Contemporary Surgical Clerkships

AF147569

Series Editor
Adam E. M. Eltorai, Marlborough, MA, USA

This series of specialty-specific books will serve as high-yield, quick-reference reviews specifically for the numerous third- and fourth-year medical students rotating on surgical clerkships. Edited by experts in the field, each book includes concise review content from a senior resident or fellow and an established academic physician. Students can read the text from cover to cover to gain a general foundation of knowledge that can be built upon when they begin their rotation, or they can use specific chapters to review a subspecialty before starting a new rotation or seeing a patient with a subspecialty attending.

These books will be the ideal, on-the-spot references for medical students and practitioners seeking fast facts on diagnosis and management. Their bullet-pointed format, including user-friendly figures, tables and algorithms, make them the perfect quick-reference. Their content breadth covers the most commonly encountered problems in practice, focusing on the fundamental principles of diagnosis and management. Carry them in your white coat for convenient access to the answers you need, when you need them.

Emily Li • Colin Bacorn

Editors

Ophthalmology Clerkship

A Guide for Senior Medical Students

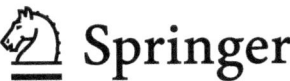 Springer

Editors
Emily Li
Wilmer Eye Institute
Johns Hopkins University
Baltimore, MD, USA

Colin Bacorn
Wilmer Eye Institute
Johns Hopkins University
Baltimore, MD, USA

ISSN 2730-941X ISSN 2730-9428 (electronic)
Contemporary Surgical Clerkships
ISBN 978-3-031-27326-1 ISBN 978-3-031-27327-8 (eBook)
https://doi.org/10.1007/978-3-031-27327-8

This Springer imprint is published by the registered company Springer Nature Switzerland AG
The registered company address is: Gewerbestrasse 11, 6330 Cham, Switzerland

Preface

Ophthalmology, the study of disease and surgery of the eye and visual systems, is an intricate and rewarding field with direct impact on patients. Pathology of the eye and periorbita significantly impacts patients' activities of daily living and quality of life and is associated with a variety of systemic conditions including infections, malignancies, and metabolic derangements. As a result, an understanding of the fundamentals of ophthalmic physiology and disease processes is beneficial to physician trainees of all persuasions.

The following compilation introduces and summarizes the ophthalmic anatomy, examination, and clinical evaluation. The material begins with an overview of ocular anatomy, which is closely entwined with visual function, and a brief discussion of optics. The remainder of the text is organized into traditional ophthalmic sub-specialties, some of which may be defined anatomically (i.e., cornea and retina) while others focus on a specific pathophysiology (i.e., glaucoma or uveitis). Oculoplastics and neuro-ophthalmology encompass the study of the structures surrounding and supporting the eye itself. Overlap in content among these chapters reflects the interplay of ophthalmic anatomy and physiology among sub-specialties and highlights each discipline's unique perspective and considerations.

Ophthalmologic annotation makes frequent use of esoteric jargon and abbreviations not commonly shared with other medical specialties. This unique terminology can be an obstacle to students first studying ophthalmology. The text discusses and defines specialty-specific terms as they become relevant so that students can develop a familiarity with the language commonly encountered on an ophthalmology rotation.

We hope that the following text serves as a practical companion to your ophthalmology clerkship and provides an immersive introduction that inspires further learning.

Baltimore, MD, USA   Emily Li
Baltimore, MD, USA   Colin Bacorn

Contents

Abbreviations

AAION	Arteritic anterior ischemic optic neuropathy
AC	Anterior chamber
ACG	Angle closure glaucoma
ACIOL	Anterior chamber intraocular lens
ALT	Argon laser trabeculoplasty
AMD	Age-related macular degeneration, also ARMD
ARN	Acute retinal necrosis
ARx	Autorefraction
ATs	Artificial tears
BCL	Bandage contact lens
Bleph	Blepharoplasty, alternatively blepharitis
BRAO	Branch retinal artery occlusion
BRVO	Branch retinal vein occlusion
C/D	Cup-to-disc ratio, also C:D
C/S	Conjunctiva and sclera
CB	Ciliary body
CCT	Central corneal thickness
cDCR	Conjunctivodacryocystorhinostomy, surgical procedure
CEIOL	Cataract extraction with insertion of intraocular lens
CF	Count fingers, quantification of visual acuity
CME	Cystoid macular edema
CNV	Choroidal neovascularization
CPC	Cyclophotocoagulation, glaucoma procedure
CRAO	Central retinal artery occlusion
CRVO	Central retinal vein occlusion
CSM	Central steady and maintained, quantification of visual acuity
CWS	Cotton wool spot
DALK	Deep anterior lamellar keratoplasty
DBH	Dot-blot hemorrhage, retinal finding in diabetes
DCR	Dacryocystorhinostomy, surgical procedure
DES	Dry eye syndrome

DFE	Dilated fundus exam
DMEK	Descemet membrane endothelial keratoplasty
DSEK	Descemet's stripping endothelial keratoplasty
DVD	Dissociated vertical deviation
E	Esophoria
ECP	Endoscopic cytophocoagulation, glaucoma procedure
EL	Endolaser
ELA	External levator advancement, surgical procedure
EOM	Extraocular motility, extraocular muscle
ERG	Electroretinogram
ERM	Epiretinal membrane
ET	Esotropia
EUA	Examination under anesthesia
FA	Fluorescein angiography
FB	Foreign body
GA	Geographic atrophy
GCL	Ganglion cell layer
GDD	Glaucoma drainage device
Globe	Open globe injury
Gtt	Eye drop
HM	Hand motion, quantification of visual acuity
HSV	Herpes simplex virus
HVF	Humphrey visual field
ICG	Indocyanin green angiography
IOFB	Intraocular foreign body
IOL	Intraocular lens
IOP	Intraocular pressure
K	Cornea
KCN	Keratoconus
KNV	Corneal neovascularization
KP	Keratic precipitate
L/L	Lids and lashes
LASIK	Laser in situ keratomileusis
LF	Levator function
LL	Lower lid
LP	Light perception, quantification of visual acuity
LPI	Laser peripheral iridotomy
LTS	Lateral tarsal strip, surgical procedure
MA	Microaneurysm, retinal finding in diabetes
MGD	Meibomian gland dysfunction
MIGS	Minimally invasive glaucoma surgery
MMC	Mitomycin-c
MMCR	Muller's muscle conjunctival resection, surgical procedure
MMP	Mucus membrane pemphigoid
MRD	Margin to reflex

MRx	Manifest refraction
NAAION	Non-arteritic anterior ischemic optic neuropathy
NLDO	Nasolacrimal duct obstruction
NLP	No light perception, quantification of visual acuity
NPDR	Non-proliferative diabetic retinopathy
NS	Nuclear sclerosis, type of cataract
NVD	Neovascularization of the disc
NVG	Neovascular glaucoma
NVI	Neovascularization of the iris
OCP	Ocular cicatricial pemphigoid
OCT	Optical coherence tomography
OD	Right eye
OHTN	Ocular hypertension
OS	Left eye
OU	Both eyes
PAS	Peripheral anterior synechiae
PCIOL	Posterior chamber intraocular lens
PCO	Posterior capsular opacity
PD	Pupillary distance
PDR	Proliferative diabetic retinopathy
PDT	Photodynamic therapy
PEE	Punctate epithelial erosions
PF	Prednisolone acetate ("pred forte")
PFATs	Preservative-free artificial tears
ph	Pinhole test
Phaco	Phacoemulsification
PI	Peripheral iridotomy
PK	Penetrating keratoplasty, see also PKP
PKP	Penetrating keratoplasty, see also PK
plano	No refractive power
POAG	Primary open-angle glaucoma
POHS	Presumed ocular histoplasmosis
PORN	Peripheral outer retinal necrosis
PPA	Peripapillary atrophy
PPV	Pars plana vitrectomy, surgical procedure
PRK	Photorefractive keratectomy
PRP	Panretinal photocoagulation
PSC	Posterior subcapsular cataract
PVD	Posterior vitreous detachment
rAPD	Relative afferent pupillary defect
RB	Retinoblastoma
RD	Retinal detachment
RGP	Rigid gas-permeable contact lens
RNFL	Retinal nerve fiber layer
ROP	Retinopathy of prematurity

RP	Retinitis pigmentosa
RPE	Retinal pigment epithelium
SB	Scleral buckle
SLE	Slit lamp examination
SLT	Selective laser trabeculoplasty
SO	Silicone oil, alternatively superior oblique
Sphere	No astigmatic correction
SPK	Superficial punctate keratopathy
TBUT	Tear breakup time
TED	Thyroid eye disease
TM	Trabecular meshwork
Trab	Trabeculectomy, surgical procedure
TRD	Tractional retinal detachment
Tube	Glaucoma drainage device
UL	Upper lid
Ung	Ointment
VA	Visual acuity
VAcc	Vision with correction (glasses)
VAsc	Vision without correction (no glasses)
VZV	Varicella zoster virus
X	Exophoria
XT	Exotropia
YAG	Laser type, also name of procedure

Contributors

Tessnim R. Ahmad, MD Department of Ophthalmology, University of California, San Francisco, San Francisco, CA, USA

Colin Bacorn, MD Wilmer Eye Institute, Johns Hopkins University, Baltimore, MD, USA

Elizabeth Bolton, MD Department of Ophthalmology, Northwestern University Feinberg School of Medicine, Chicago, IL, USA

Anh D. Bui, MD, PhD Department of Ophthalmology, University of California, San Francisco, San Francisco, CA, USA

Stephanie P. Chen, MD Department of Ophthalmology, University of California, San Francisco, San Francisco, CA, USA

Lauren Collwell, MD Department of Ophthalmology and Visual Sciences, University of Massachusetts Chan Medical School, Worcester, MA, USA

Alberto Distefano, MD Department of Ophthalmology, Boston University School of Medicine, Boston, MA, USA

Jacob S. Heng, MD, PhD Department of Ophthalmology and Visual Science, Yale School of Medicine, New Haven, CT, USA

Laura C. Huang Department of Ophthalmology, Seattle Children's Hospital and University of Washington, Seattle, WA, USA

Russell Huang, MD Department of Ophthalmology, Northwestern University Feinberg School of Medicine, Chicago, IL, USA

Christopher J. Hwang, MD, MPH Department of Ophthalmology, University of North Carolina at Chapel Hill, Chapel Hill, NC, USA

Karen Jeng-Miller, MD, MPH Department of Ophthalmology and Visual Sciences, University of Massachusetts Chan Medical School, Worcester, MA, USA

J. Minjy Kang, MD Department of Ophthalmology, Northwestern University Feinberg School of Medicine, Chicago, IL, USA

Ninani Kombo, MD Department of Ophthalmology and Visual Science, Yale School of Medicine, New Haven, CT, USA

Samuel Kushner-Lenhoff Department of Ophthalmology, University of Washington, Seattle, WA, USA

Emily Li, MD Wilmer Eye Institute, Johns Hopkins University, Baltimore, MD, USA

Rebecca Li, MD Department of Ophthalmology, University of North Carolina at Chapel Hill, Chapel Hill, NC, USA

Nicole R. Mattson Department of Ophthalmology, University of Washington, Seattle, WA, USA

Charles Miller, BA Department of Ophthalmology, Northwestern University Feinberg School of Medicine, Chicago, IL, USA

Hannah Miller, MD Department of Ophthalmology, University of North Carolina at Chapel Hill, Chapel Hill, NC, USA

Neel D. Pasricha, MD Department of Ophthalmology, University of California, San Francisco, San Francisco, CA, USA

Lindsay Rothfield, MD Department of Ophthalmology, Boston University School of Medicine, Boston, MA, USA

N. Maxwell Scoville Department of Ophthalmology, University of Washington, Seattle, WA, USA

Grace L. Su Department of Ophthalmology, Seattle Children's Hospital and University of Washington, Seattle, WA, USA

Emily K. Tam Department of Ophthalmology, Seattle Children's Hospital and University of Washington, Seattle, WA, USA

Sean Teebagy, BA Department of Ophthalmology and Visual Sciences, University of Massachusetts Chan Medical School, Worcester, MA, USA

Alexandra Van Brummen Department of Ophthalmology, University of Washington, Seattle, WA, USA

Catherine Wang, BS The Johns Hopkins University School of Medicine, Baltimore, MD, USA

Jia Xu, MD Department of Ophthalmology, Boston University School of Medicine, Boston, MA, USA

Sidra Zafar, MD Wilmer Eye Institute, Johns Hopkins Hospital, Baltimore, MD, USA

Xiyu Zhao, BS The Johns Hopkins University School of Medicine, Baltimore, MD, USA

Chapter 1
Overview of Anatomy

Colin Bacorn and Emily Li

Ocular Adnexa [1, 2]

Eyelid

There are four eyelids which serve to protect the globe and help maintain vision. The upper eyelid begins at the superior orbital rim below the thicker skin of the brow and terminates at the **lid margin** from which lashes emanate. Similarly, the lower lid begins at the inferior orbital rim and extends superiorly to a corresponding lid margin. The distance between the upper and lower eyelid margins is known as the **vertical palpebral fissure**. Both eyelids are anchored medially and laterally to the bony orbit by the medial and lateral **canthal tendons.** The distance between the medial and lateral canthal angles is known as the **horizontal palpebral fissure**.

- The eyelids are composite structures with a lamellar arrangement of skin, muscle, connective tissue, fat, and **conjunctiva.** This cross-sectional anatomy is complex and changes as one progresses superiorly from the lid margin to the brow (Fig. 1.1)

    – At the level of the tarsus, the tissues are arranged from superficial to deep:

    > Skin, orbicularis oculi, tarsus, conjunctiva

    – Additional structures are present superior to the tarsus and are arranged:

    > Skin, orbicularis, septum, pre-aponeurotic fat, levator aponeurosis, Müller's muscle, and conjunctiva

C. Bacorn · E. Li (✉)
Wilmer Eye Institute, Johns Hopkins University, Baltimore, MD, USA
e-mail: cbacorn1@jh.edu; eli20@jhmi.edu

E. Li, C. Bacorn (eds.), *Ophthalmology Clerkship*, Contemporary Surgical Clerkships, https://doi.org/10.1007/978-3-031-27327-8_1

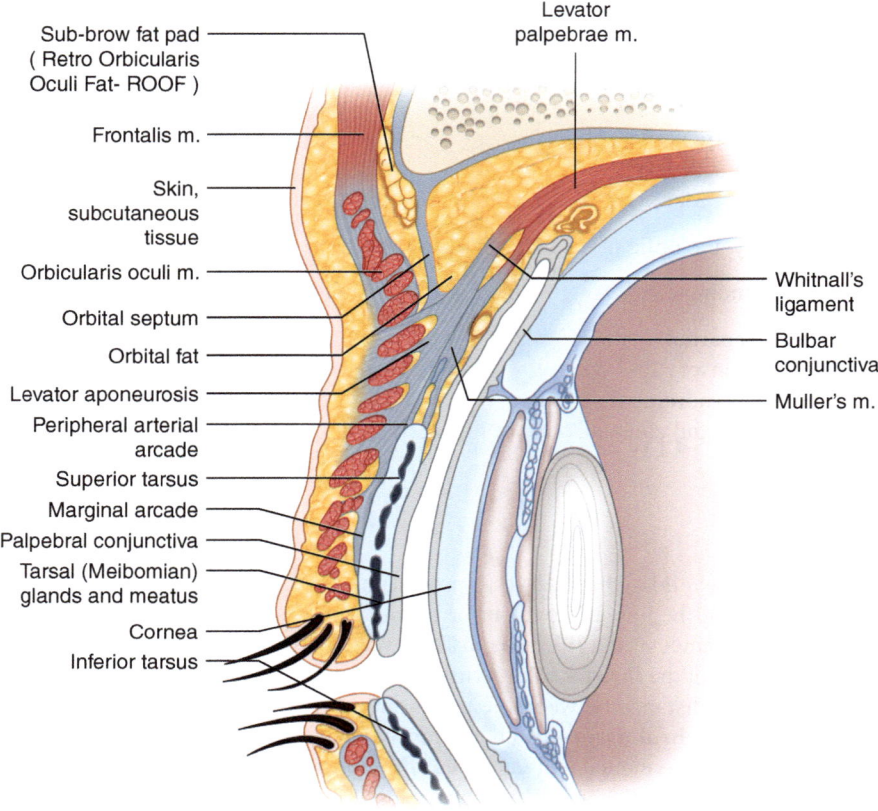

Fig. 1.1 Anatomy of the upper eyelid in cross section highlighting the anterior lamella (skin and orbicularis) as well as the posterior lamella (tarsus and conjunctiva). The major eyelid elevators, the levator palpebrae and Muller's muscle are present superior to the tarsus and deep to the orbital septum. (Source: Wolters Kluwer Health)

- **Tarsus** (tarsal plate)—rigid structure that provides mechanical integrity to the lid
- **Septum**—fibrous sheet extending from the orbital rim to the tarsus

    Important surgical landmark
    Barrier preventing spread of superficial (**pre-septal**) infections to deeper orbital structures (**orbital cellulitis**)

- Several distinct muscles are responsible for the movement of the eyelids:

    - **Orbicularis oculi**—annular subcutaneous protractor to close the upper and lower lids, innervated by the facial nerve

- **Levator palpebrae superioris**—responsible for retraction, or elevation, of the upper eyelid, innervated by oculomotor nerve
- Superior tarsal (**Müller's**) muscle—lesser contribution to upper lid elevation, sympathetic innervation
- **Capsulopalpebral fascia** and **inferior tarsal muscle**—lower lid analogs of the levator and Müller's muscles

    Less distinct and are difficult to distinguish from one another surgically; often referred to collectively as the **lower lid retractors**

- The eyelids have three primary functions:

  - Mechanical protection
  - Lubrication

      Contain meibomian glands and accessory lacrimal glands which secrete components of the tear film

      - **Meibomian glands**—located in the tarsus, secret the oil component of tears through orifices at the lid margin

  - Clearance of tears and foreign debris from the ocular surface

Nasolacrimal System

The air-tear film interface is the major refracting interface of the eye and plays an important role in vision. The tear film coats the ocular surface, prevents the accumulation of foreign material and pathogens, and helps maintain health of the anterior eye. Disorders of the tear film or blockages of tear clearance are common causes of functional impairment and serious eye disorders up to and including blindness.

- **Lacrimal glands**—exocrine glands located in the superolateral orbit; primary site of tear production.
- Tears drain through the **puncta** (orifices in the margin of the medial upper and lower lid) into the canaliculus, **lacrimal sac,** and nasolacrimal duct before ultimately reaching the nose (Fig. 1.2)

  - Obstructions along this path may result in **epiphora** (tearing)
  - Students should be careful not to confuse the terms for inflammation/infection of the lacrimal *gland* (**dacryoadenitis**) with inflammation/infection of the lacrimal *sac* (**dacryocystitis**)

Fig. 1.2 Nasolacrimal
system anatomy.
[Reproduced from Ducker
et al. [4] under Creative
Commons Attribution
License 4.0 (Source:
Ducker L, Rivera
RY. Anatomy, Head and
Neck, Eye Lacrimal Duct.
[Updated 2021 Aug 11].
In: StatPearls [Internet].
Treasure Island (FL):
StatPearls Publishing;
2022 Jan. Available from:
https://www.ncbi.nlm.nih.
gov/books/NBK531487/)]

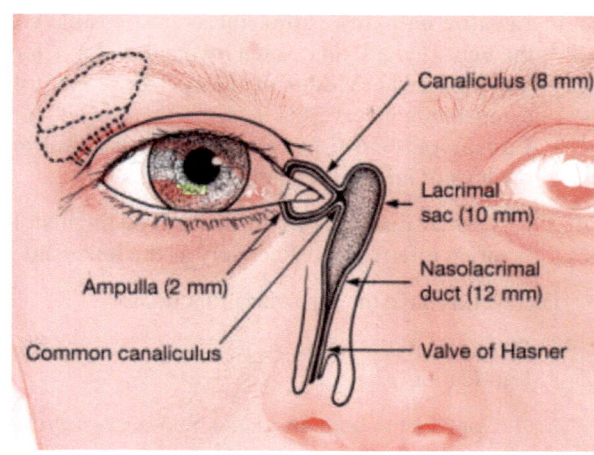

Orbit [1, 2]

The orbit is a pear-shaped cavity formed by the bones of the skull and face and enclosed anteriorly by the orbital septum. The orbit houses the globe along with its associated muscles, vasculature, nerves, and lymphatic drainage system. Most structures enter the orbit through foramina at its posterior extent (**apex**). Due to its bony walls, and the inelastic septum at its anterior aperture, the volume of the orbit is fixed at 30 cm^3. This anatomic feature has important clinical repercussions as space-occupying processes in the orbit may cause permanent compressive vision loss.

Bones

Seven bones articulate to form the medial wall, floor, lateral wall, and roof of the orbit (Fig. 1.3). These bones and the contents of the foramina passing through them should be committed to memory as they are frequently affected by trauma and are helpful in localizing orbital pathology.

- The medial wall is composed of the **sphenoid**, **maxillary**, **ethmoid,** and **lacrimal** bones
    - Thinnest wall of the orbit, commonly fractured in trauma
    - Anterior and posterior **ethmoidal foramina** transmit their respective **arteries**

        Important surgical landmarks and potential conduits for infection to spread from the ethmoid sinus into the orbit
- The orbital floor is composed of the **palatine**, sphenoid, and maxillary bones

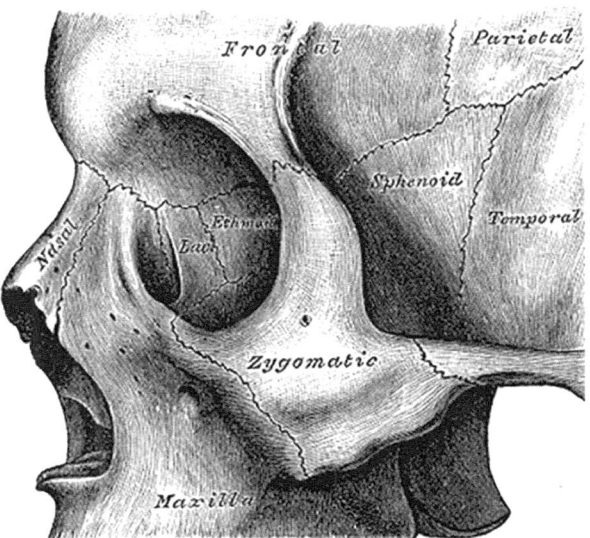

Fig. 1.3 Oblique view demonstrating bony anatomy of the left orbit; [5] see also Fig. 1.1 of oculoplastics chapter. Note that a small component of the posterior orbital floor is composed of the palatine bone which is not visible in this oblique view. (Source: Gray, Henry. *Anatomy of the Human Body.* Philadelphia: Lea & Febiger, 1918)

- **Infraorbital canal** of the floor contains the **infraorbital nerve** (branch of V_2)

    Damage leads to hypoesthesia of the ipsilateral cheek, lip, and gum

- Bone is thinnest adjacent to the infraorbital canal and fractures are common

    "Blow-out" fracture—fracture of the orbital floor with an intact orbital rim

• The lateral wall is composed of the sphenoid and **zygomatic** bones

- A particularly sturdy vertical buttress supporting the face

    Less frequently fractured and has relatively few perforating vessels and nerves

• The orbital roof is composed of the **frontal** and sphenoid bones.

- Separates the orbit from the frontal sinus (anteriorly) or the cranial fossa (posteriorly)

    Fractures of the roof are less common
    Posterior roof fractures warrant neurosurgical evaluation

The posterior extent of the orbit is known as the apex and contains the **superior** and **inferior orbital fissures,** as well as the **optic canal**. Many of the extraocular muscles have a common origin at the apex (**Annulus of Zinn**), which serves to divide the orbit into **intraconal** and **extraconal** compartments (the term "-conal" refers to the muscle cone extending from the annulus to the muscle insertions on the globe which will be discussed later in this chapter).

- Nerves passing into the orbit from the cavernous sinus traverse the superior orbital fissure.

  - **Oculomotor**, nasociliary (branch of V_1), and **abducens nerves** pass within the Annulus of Zinn
  - **Trochlear**, lacrimal, and frontal nerves (branches of V_1) pass outside of the Annulus of Zinn.

    As a result, unaffected by local anesthetics administered as a retrobulbar block

- The inferior orbital fissure does not communicate with the cavernous sinus or intracranial space and, compared to the superior fissure, transmits fewer structures.
- The **optic nerve** runs through the optic canal as it leaves the orbit and travels posteriorly to the chiasm.

  - Part of the central nervous system and all three meningeal layers and myelinated after exiting the globe.

    Susceptible to increases in intracranial pressure as well as demyelinating disease

  - The orbital portion of the optic nerve is longer than necessary to bridge the distance from the posterior **sclera** to the optic canal

    Redundancy allows for movement and anterior displacement of the globe (**proptosis**) without damaging the nerve

  - Penetrated by the **central retinal artery** (a branch of the ophthalmic artery), the primary blood supply of the inner retina

Extraocular Muscles

There are six extraocular muscles in the orbit responsible for movement of the globe. These are the **medial, inferior, lateral,** and **superior recti muscles** and the **superior** and **inferior oblique muscles** (Fig. 1.4a, b). The four recti muscles have a common origin at the apex called the Annulus of Zinn and divide the orbit into intraconal and extraconal spaces. Additional extraocular muscles include the upper eyelid retractors (the previously mentioned levator and Müller's muscle) and their lower eyelid analogs (the capsulopalpebral fascia and inferior tarsal muscle).

- The medial rectus is innervated by the oculomotor nerve and is responsible for adduction.
- The lateral rectus is innervated by the abducens nerve and is responsible for abduction.
- The superior rectus is innervated by the oculomotor nerve and is responsible for supraduction (as well as adduction and incyclotorsion).

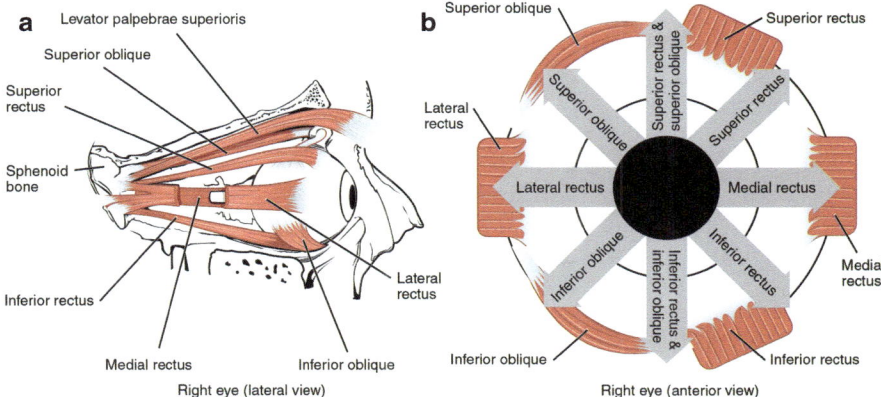

Fig. 1.4 Extraocular muscle anatomy and actions. (Reproduced from OpenStax [6] under Creative Commons Attribution License 4.0. Access for free at https://openstax.org/books/anatomy-and-physiology/pages/1-introduction)

- The inferior rectus is innervated by the oculomotor nerve and is responsible for infraduction (as well as adduction and excyclotorsion).
- The superior oblique is innervated by the trochlear nerve and is responsible for incyclotorsion (as well as infraduction and abduction).

    - Originates at the orbital apex (superior to the Annulus of Zinn), courses anteriorly to the cartilaginous **trochlea** where it is redirected laterally to insert onto the sclera

- The inferior oblique is innervated by the oculomotor nerve and is responsible for excyclotorsion (as well as supraduction and abduction).

    - Originates on the medial aspect of the orbital floor, runs laterally to insert onto the sclera

- The recti muscles each have anterior tendinous portions which insert into the sclera several millimeters posterior to the corneal **limbus**.

    - Allow for motility and carry important blood supply (**anterior ciliary arteries**) to the anterior portion of the globe
    - Medial rectus inserts closest to the limbus followed by the inferior, lateral and superior recti muscles; a relationship named the **Spiral of Tillaux**

Globe [2]

The globe is responsible for collecting, focusing, and initial processing of light information to allow for sight. It is an incredibly complex organ with numerous interacting subsystems. While examining and operating on the globe requires

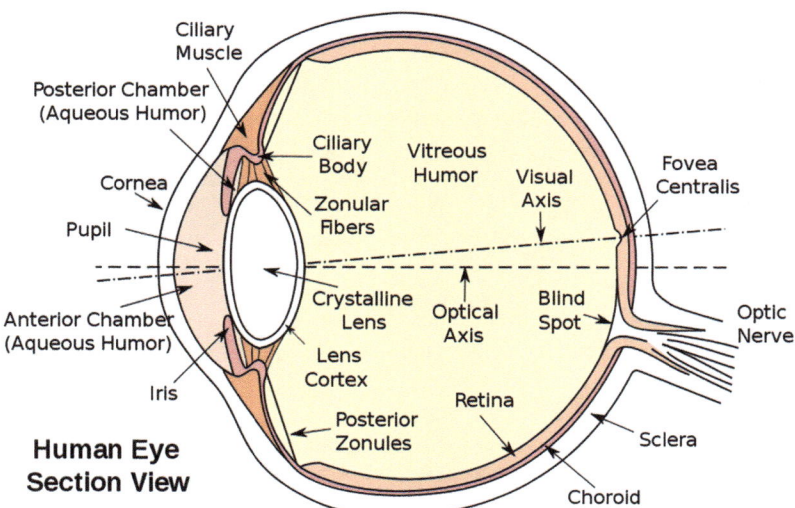

Fig. 1.5 Anatomy of the globe demonstrating the outer coats of the eye (sclera, uvea, retina) as well as the major structures of the anterior and posterior segments. Public domain material reproduced from Wikimedia Commons. (Source: ZStardust B. *Section View of the Human Eye. Based on Image:Eyesection.Gif.*; 2007. Accessed July 20, 2022. https://commons.wikimedia.org/wiki/File:Eyesection.svg)

delicacy and precision, you will be surprised by its paradoxical resilience and the ability to withstand and recover from trauma. It is conceptually useful to highlight the three concentric coats of the wall of the globe; an outer coat of **cornea** and sclera, a middle coat of **uvea** (**iris**, **ciliary body** and **choroid**) and an inner coat of **retina**. A second useful classification is the division of the globe into an **anterior segment** (cornea, iris, ciliary body and lens) and a **posterior segment** (**vitreous humor**, retina, choroid, and optic nerve head). These classifications are complementary and not mutually exclusive (Fig. 1.5). While the globe proper is confined by the cornea and sclera, the overlying **conjunctiva** and **Tenon's capsule** are intimately associated with a large portion of this surface and warrant comment here.

Conjunctiva

The conjunctiva is the mucosal lining which covers the anterior portion of the globe (except the cornea) and the inner surface of the eyelids. It is tightly adherent at the limbus and becomes progressively less closely associated with the globe as it travels posteriorly until it fully separates and reflects anteriorly upon itself to line the lids. In this arrangement, the **palpebral conjunctiva** of the lid is in direct apposition with the **bulbar conjunctiva** of the globe; the potential space between these two surfaces is the **fornix.**

- Contains numerous mucin secreting goblet cells; lubricates the ocular surface
- **Symblepharon**—abnormal adhesions of the bulbar and palpebral conjunctiva
- **Ankyloblepharon**—abnormal fusion of the upper and lower palpebral conjunctiva bridging the palpebral fissure

Tenon's Capsule

Lying deep to the conjunctiva, Tenon's capsule invests the globe from the limbus to optic nerve. Where it is pierced by the extraocular muscles it reflects posteriorly and coats the muscle tendons to contribute to the intermuscular septum.

- Important barrier preventing orbital fat from prolapsing anteriorly over the globe beneath the conjunctiva

  - Violation during surgery can lead to fat adherence and restrictive scarring

Sclera

The sclera is the outer shell encapsulating the intraocular contents and runs from the optic nerve at its **posterior pole** an anterior orifice that is vaulted by the cornea. Comprised of type 1 collagen, the tough sclera maintains the normal shape of the globe and is an effective barrier to penetrating injury, as well as infectious, thermal, and chemical insults to the globe.

- The **limbus** is the anterior boundary of the sclera and divides the sclera and cornea.

  - Site of tightest adherence and fusion of conjunctiva and Tenon's capsule

- Scleral thickness varies from 1 mm at the posterior pole near the insertion of the optic nerve to 0.3 mm just posterior to extraocular muscle insertions.

  - The muscle insertions are common locations for scleral rupture

- The sclera is perforated by the optic nerve posteriorly and has multiple smaller perforations for the **anterior** and **posterior ciliary arteries** and the **vortex veins**.

Cornea

The clear anterior projection of the globe, through which the colored iris is visible, is called the cornea. Bounded by the limbus, the cornea averages 11.5 mm in diameter in adults and is steeper and thinner centrally than it is peripherally (prolate in shape). The cornea has five distinct anatomic layers which contribute to its optical and mechanical properties (epithelium, **Bowman's layer**, stroma, **Descemet's membrane**, and endothelium).

- The cornea's clarity is a result of:
  - Precise arrangement of type 1 collagen fibers in the **stroma**
  - Constant pump action of the **endothelium** preventing fluid accumulation and swelling
- The cornea is avascular and supplied with oxygen and nutrients from the tear film externally and the aqueous humor internally
  - Key factor in **immune privilege** and the success of corneal transplantation
- The **long ciliary nerves** (branches of V_1) run anteriorly between the sclera and choroid before terminating in the cornea to provide a rich sensory innervation.
  - Explains the severe pain associated with corneal abrasions
  - Essential for the health of the cornea; loss of corneal sensation can lead to corneal opacification and blindness

Anterior Chamber

Deep to the cornea and anterior to the iris is a fluid-filled space called the **anterior chamber**. **Aqueous humor**, the fluid, is produced by the ciliary body and enters the anterior chamber through the pupil before draining into the **trabecular meshwork**. The trabecular meshwork is an intricate structure located at the periphery of the anterior chamber adjacent to the limbus and will be discussed in more detail in the glaucoma chapter of this text.

- The anterior chamber can become opaque in a variety of pathologic processes.
  - **Hyphema**—the accumulation of red blood cells in the anterior chamber
  - **Hypopyon**—layering of white blood cells inferiorly
  - Either type of **cell** or small amounts of protein ("**flare**") can be quantified at the slit lamp

Uvea

The term uvea refers to the iris, ciliary body, and choroid. They form the contiguous middle coat of the globe's lining. These structures are highly vascularized and prone to inflammation, which will be discussed in more detail in the uveitis chapter.

- The iris is an annular, pigmented structure posterior to the anterior chamber.
  - Blocks off-axis and scattered light rays to increase the clarity of vision.

    Long ciliary nerves (sympathetic) activate the radially oriented **iris dilator** muscle dilate the pupil

Short ciliary nerves (parasympathetic) activate the circumferential **iris sphincter** to constrict the pupil

- The ciliary body is located posterior to the iris and anterior to the vitreous at the **ora serrata**. It is tightly adherent to the sclera and has several distinct muscle layers covered by a double layer of epithelium arranged into folds called **ciliary processes**. This complex structure allows the ciliary body to serve two primary functions:

  - Epithelium of ciliary processes produces aqueous humor and drives the intra-ocular pressure
  - Changes in the tension of the muscles are transmitted through the **zonules** to the lens to adjust its position and shape

    Alters refractive power and focal length of the eye

- The most posterior component of the uvea is the choroid, which lies between the outer retina and the sclera.

  - Highly vascularized structure consisting of layers of branching and looping vessels supplied by the posterior ciliary arteries.
  - High perfusion provides oxygen and nutrients to, and carries waste away from, the metabolically active photoreceptors and outer retina.
  - **Bruch's membrane**—innermost layer of the choroid, functions as an important physical barrier preventing abnormal vessel growth beneath the retina.

Lens

The crystalline lens rests posterior to the iris and has several distinct layers. The outermost layer is the capsule. The capsule is the basement membrane of the second layer, the metabolically active lens epithelium. Lens fibers, cells that have matured from epithelial cells and lost their nuclei, are deep into the epithelium. They are arrayed in tightly packed concentric layers and form the bulk of the lens. This entire structure is suspended by a radial arrangement of zonules connecting the lens equator to the ciliary body. Constriction of the ciliary body relaxes the radial tension of the zonules and allows the central anterior-posterior thickness of the lens to increase. This increases the refractive power of the eye and brings near objects into focus (**accommodation**). Conversely, when the ciliary body relaxes, zonular tension increases and the lens shape is altered so that light from distant objects is focused on the retina.

- Contributes roughly one third of the refractive power of the eye.
- The lens grows throughout life as additional lens fibers form.

  - Causes a loss of optical clarity (**cataract** formation) and increased rigidity/loss of accommodation (**presbyopia**).

Vitreous

The vitreous humor, a largely acellular loose matrix of collagen fibrils, makes up the bulk of the volume of the posterior segment and overall globe (4.5 mL out of 6 mL total). The vitreous, by virtue of its volume, maintains the shape of the globe. It is most tightly adherent to the inner coats of the globe anteriorly at the ora serrata (the **vitreous base**) and posteriorly at the optic nerve head, as well as along retinal blood vessels.

- Degenerates and liquifies with age; as the collagen matrix breaks down, or as a result of trauma, the vitreous may detach from the retina.
    - Generally has no permanent effect on vision but occasionally associated with retinal tear or detachment.

Retina

The innermost lining of the globe is the retina, the photosensitive tissue of the eye. It is composed of ten highly specialized layers that transmit light information to the optic nerve and ultimately to the occipital cortex of the brain. Light passes through the retina and is detected by **photoreceptors** in the outermost layer of the retina before nervous impulses are transmitted back inward to the **ganglion cell layer**. The ganglion cell layer consists of the cell bodies of the neurons whose axons converge at the optic disc and exit the posterior sclera to form the optic nerve.

- Photoreceptors classified as **rods** or **cones**
    - Rods greatly outnumber cones and are more sensitive to faint light stimuli
    - Cones specialized to detect color and motion; three subtypes

The retina has dual blood supply from the central retinal arty (inner one third of the retina) and the choroid (outer two third). The central retinal artery enters the globe in the center of the optic nerve and branches into four arcades (two nasal and two temporal) before coursing peripherally in the plane between the retina and the vitreous.

- Temporal arcades border the macula superiorly and inferiorly; important clinical and surgical landmarks for identifying the extent of the macula
- Blood returns from the inner retina along venous arcades which the mirror courses of the arterial arcades
    - Converge on the optic nerve head exit the globe alongside the central retinal artery as the **central retinal vein**

In addition to this "inside–outside" structural organization, the retina also has important anatomic variation radially as it proceeds from center to periphery. The posterior most portion of the retina is the **macula**, which processes light for central vision. The remainder of the retina extends anteriorly along the inner surface of the globe in all directions to terminate at the ora serrata.

- **Fovea**—avascular center of the macula; greatest density of cones found in the retina

  - Provides high acuity central fixation

- Peripherally cone density rapidly decreases and rods predominate beyond the macula

Introduction to Clinical Optics [3]

Understanding the function of the eye requires a basic understanding of how light interacts with the optical media of the eye and properties of light itself. While in reality, light has properties of both a wave and a particle, it is more convenient for the ophthalmologist to treat light geometrically as an idealized **ray**. In this paradigm, light is emitted from a point source and passes through the clear structures of the globe before reaching the retina.

When a ray of light crosses from one media to another, for instance, from the aqueous humor to the crystalline lens, the angle at which it crosses this interface (the angle of incidence) and the refractive indices of both media determine the behavior of the light ray.

- **Angle of incidence** (θ)—angle between a ray of light and the interface it crosses
- **Refractive index** (n)—material property intrinsic to a given media

If the angle of incidence is not perpendicular to the plane of the interface and the indices of refraction of the two media differ from one another, the ray of light will bend and change direction. This phenomenon is known as **refraction** and is the basis on which lens systems, including those of the eye, function.

- **Snell's law**—description of the behavior of refracted light [$n_1 \times \sin(\theta_1) = n_2 \times \sin(\theta_2)$] (Fig. 1.6)

Fig. 1.6 Visual representation of the refraction of a ray of light as it traverses the interface between materials of differing refractive indices. (Source: Oleg Alexandrov. *English: Snell's Law.*; 2006. Accessed July 20, 2022. https://commons. wikimedia.org/wiki/ File:Snells_law.svg)

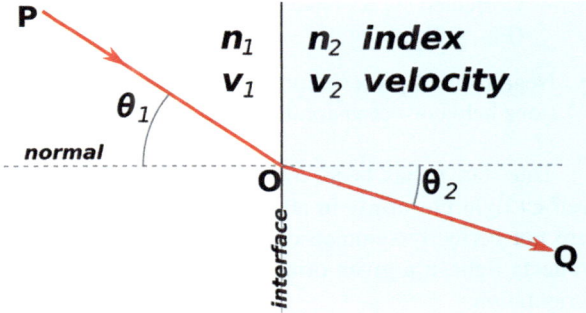

The geometry of a lens affects the behavior of light when it passes through the lens. Parallel light rays entering a **convex lens** (such as the crystalline lens in the eye) will exit the lens converging towards a **focal point**. In contrast, light rays diverge away from one another after passing through a **concave lens**.

- Focal point of a convex lens is located on the side of the *exiting* light rays and is the point at which they converge
- Focal point of a concave lens is the point from which exiting light rays appear to originate and is located on the same side of the lens as the *entering* light rays

The unit used to quantify the amount of **vergence** (convergence or divergence) of light is the **diopter** (D).

- Can be calculated as the reciprocal of **focal length** (distance from the lens to the focal point)
- More powerful lenses refract light more strongly and have shorter focal lengths (higher absolute dioptric powers)
  - By convention, converging lenses have positive dioptric power while diverging lenses have negative dioptric power.
  - For example, A + 8D lens is more powerful and bends light to a greater degree than a + 6D lens. A + 8D lens and a -8D lens have the same power and focal length, but the focal points are on opposite sides of the lens relative to one another.

As anyone who wears contacts or glasses knows, lenses can be used to correct vision. The ideal eye is **emmetropic** which means that the light from distant objects (greater than approximately 20 feet) is perfectly focused on the retina after passing through the optical media of the eye (the air-tear interface and lens). However, most eyes are not emmetropic and light will either be focused on a point anterior to the retina (i.e., in the vitreous cavity) or to a point posterior to the retina.

- **Myopia**—focal point of the eye is anterior to the retina ("near-sighted").
  - Corrected by a concave lens in front of the eye to reduce refractive power (Fig. 1.7a).
- **Hyperopia**—focal point of the eye is posterior to the retina ("far-sighted").
  - Corrected by a convex lens in front of the eye to increase refractive power (Fig. 1.7b).
- Negative lens prescriptions are for near-sighted patients, while positive prescriptions help correct vision for those who are far-sighted.

Thus far, it has been convenient to discuss lenses which are symmetric and refract light uniformly in all orientations. However, in reality, most natural lenses are not perfectly symmetric and have some **astigmatism**. In this scenario, a lens reflects light in a given orientation more strongly than light perpendicular to that orientation.

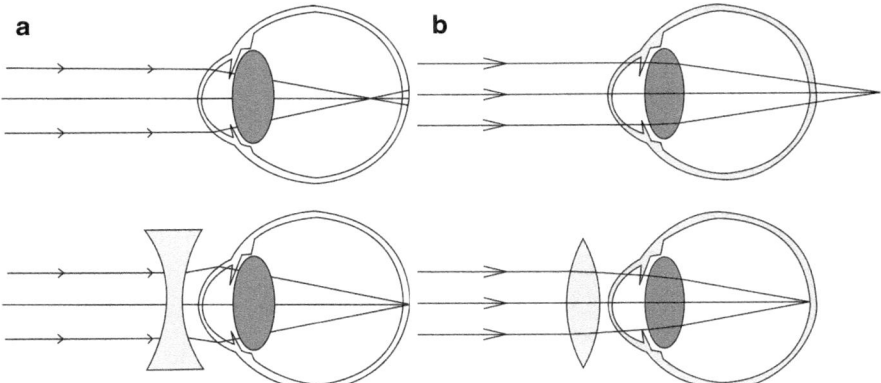

Fig. 1.7 (**a**) In a myopic eye, light rays are focused anterior to the retina, a concave lens placed in front of the eye corrects this defocus. (**b**) Conversely, in hyperopia light rays are focused posterior to the retina and a convex lens reduces the focal length so that images are focused on the retina. Public domain material reproduced from Wikimedia Commons. (7a—Source: Garantulis P. *Drawing with Shaded Lenses.*; 2010. Accessed July 20, 2022. https://commons.wikimedia.org/wiki/File:Myopia-2-3.svg/Source: CryptWizard. *English: Schematic Representation of Hypermetropia.*; 2007. Accessed July 20, 2022. https://commons.wikimedia.org/wiki/File:Hypermetropia.svg)

- Corrected by wearing glasses or contact lenses with different refractive powers in perpendicular axes

  While the use of corrective lenses is the most common technique to treat refractive error, the **pinhole** is an alternative, quick, technique routinely used during the ophthalmic examination to refine visual acuity.

- Patient asked to look through a small aperture (1.2 mm in diameter) and their visual acuity is assessed
- The pinhole blocks off-axis light rays, allowing only central rays perpendicular to the visual axis to pass through to the fovea
- Minimizes effect of myopia, hyperopia, and astigmatism up to approximately four diopters

  – Failure to improve with the pinhole test may signal ophthalmic pathology

References

1. Salmon J. Kanski's clinical ophthalmology: a systematic approach. 9th ed. Amsterdam: Elsevier Health Sciences; 2019.
2. Brar V. 2021–2022 Basic and clinical science course, section 02: fundamentals and principles of ophthalmology. San Francisco: American Academy of Ophthalmology; 2021.
3. Schwartz S. Geometrical and visual optics: a clinical introduction. 2nd ed. New York: McGraw-Hill Education; 2013.

4. Ducker L, Rivera RY. Anatomy, head and neck, eye lacrimal duct. Treasure Island (FL): StatPearls Publishing; 2022.
5. Gray H. Anatomy of the human body. Philadelphia: Lea & Febiger; 1918.
6. Ch. 1 Introduction—Anatomy and Physiology | OpenStax. https://openstax.org/books/anatomy-and-physiology/pages/1-introduction. Accessed 20 July 2022.

Chapter 2
Comprehensive Eye Exam

Xiyu Zhao, Catherine Wang, Sidra Zafar, Colin Bacorn, and Emily Li

Ocular Vital Signs

Visual Acuity

Visual acuity refers to the clarity of the examinee's vision as well as the ability to perceive minute visual details with precision. Careful visual acuity examination tests underlying optical and neural factors, such as the functional health of the retina and the brain's processing capacity for visual information.

Snellen Chart [1, 2]

Visual acuity can be measured at near (14 inches from the eye) and at distance (20 feet away). The most common assessment tool is the Snellen chart (Fig. 2.1), but others include Landolt Cs or the Tumbling E chart for patients who may not be able to read letters. The Snellen chart expresses visual acuity in fraction form. The

---

Xiyu Zhao and Catherine Wang contributed equally with all other contributors.

X. Zhao (✉) · C. Wang
The Johns Hopkins University School of Medicine, Baltimore, MD, USA
e-mail: xzhao81@jhmi.edu; cwang210@jhmi.edu

S. Zafar
Wilmer Eye Institute, Johns Hopkins Hospital, Baltimore, MD, USA

C. Bacorn · E. Li
Wilmer Eye Institute, Johns Hopkins University, Baltimore, MD, USA

© The Author(s), under exclusive license to Springer Nature Switzerland AG 2023
E. Li, C. Bacorn (eds.), *Ophthalmology Clerkship*, Contemporary Surgical Clerkships, https://doi.org/10.1007/978-3-031-27327-8_2

Fig. 2.1 Snellen Chart and associated visual acuity measurements

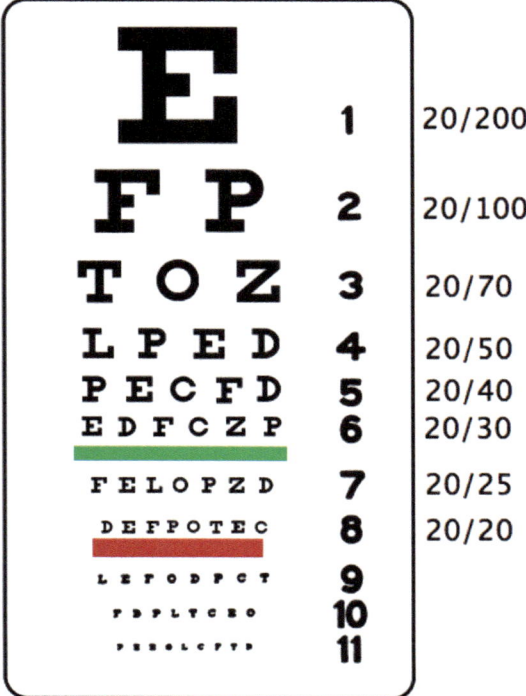

numerator refers to the distance in feet that the patients read the letters, and the denominator refers to the distance in feet that a subject with normal vision should be able to read the letters.

- Vision should be checked at one eye at a time, first with and then without spectacles, if applicable.
- Patients should be asked to identify the line of letters in the Snellen chart from left to right, top to bottom. Determine the bottommost line of which they can read a majority of the letters. Record this line as the visual acuity along with the number of letters the patient missed as a minus (i.e., 20/30 − 2) or the number of letters they can read on the next smaller line (i.e., 20/30 + 2).
- When patients' visual acuity is measured to be worse than 20/30, repeat the exam using a pinhole. An improvement in visual acuity when using a pinhole indicates that the patient's vision may improve with spectacle correction.
- If the patient is unable to read the top line of the Snellen chart, ask him or her to count fingers you hold up several feet away. Move closer to your patient until they can count fingers and record the distance.
- If the patient is unable to count fingers at 1 foot of distance, ask if the patient can sense hand motion at that distance. If the patient can sense hand motion clarify if

they can sense the direction of motion and if so, record the vision as "hand motion with direction."

- If the patient is unable to sense hand motion, test to see if the patient can determine the position of the light in quadrants. Record whether the patient has light perception with projection, light perception without projection, or no light perception. Be sure the other eye is fully occluded for accuracy.
- The "Tumbling E" chart is a tool for visual acuity assessment in young children and illiterate adults. Instead of asking the patients to identify the letters, ask them to indicate which way the letter "E" opens towards.

Pupils

Pupil testing can uncover serious retinal and neuro-ophthalmic diseases, and therefore is an integral part of every comprehensive eye examination.

Pupillary Light Reflex [2]

Pupil size is controlled by a dilator muscle (innervated by the sympathetic nervous system) and a constrictor muscle (innervated by parasympathetic fibers of cranial nerve III). Miosis refers to pupil constriction, whereas mydriasis refers to pupil dilation. Pupil size should be measured with a ruler in light and dark settings and recorded in millimeters.

- Pupillary light reflexes should be tested in one eye at a time in a dim setting. Shine a bright light into the test eye and observe for pupil constriction (Fig. 2.2a). Remove the light source and observe for pupil dilation. Repeat the test in the same eye to observe for consensual light reflex in the other eye.
- The normal state of pupils is often referred to as PERRLA (pupils equally round and reactive to light and accommodation). The accommodation reflex refers to the constriction of the pupils near focus (Fig. 2.2b). This response decreases with age.

Intraocular Pressure (IOP)

Tonometry refers to techniques used to determine the intraocular pressure. Intraocular pressure is typically reported in millimeters of mercury (mmHg). It can help detect ocular hypertension, seen in conditions such as glaucoma and uveitis, and ocular hypotension, seen with postoperative wound leaks and perforations of the globe.

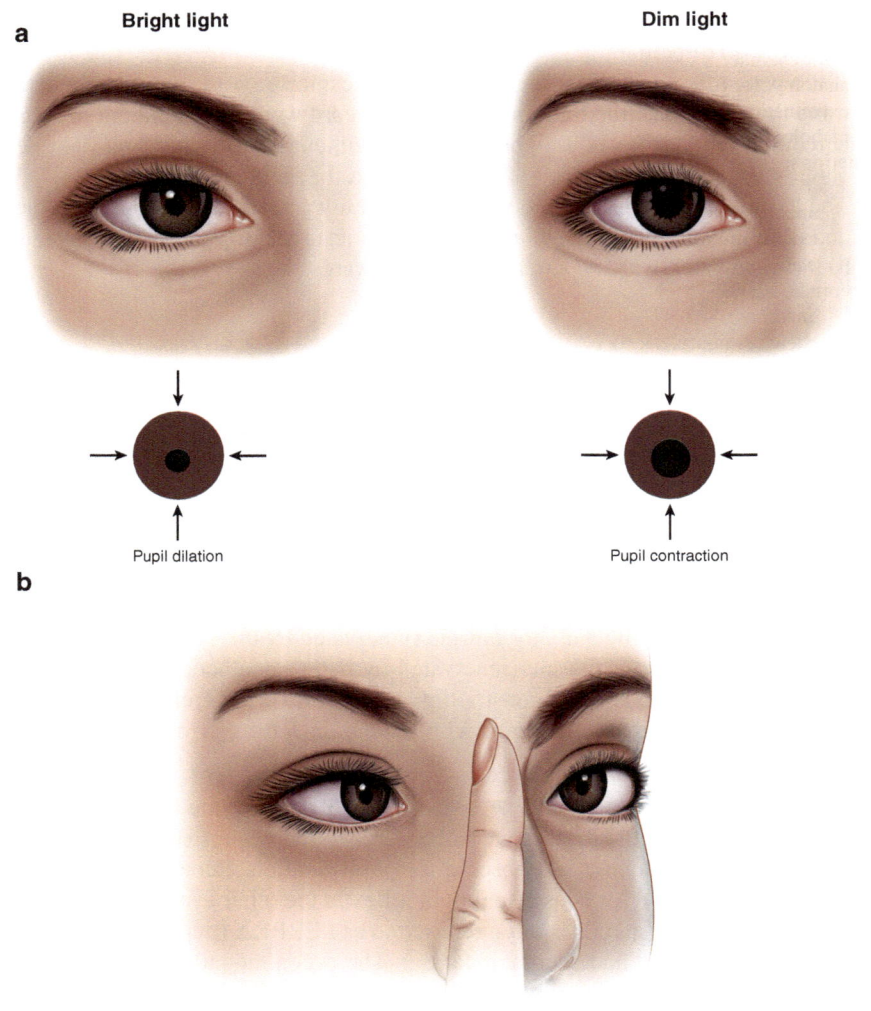

Fig. 2.2 (**a**) Demonstration of pupillary light reflex under bright light and dim light. (**b**) Demonstration of accommodation reflex. Pupils should constrict when focused on closer objects

- Tonometers may be divided into two main categories: applanation and indentation tonometers. Applanation tonometers measure intraocular pressure based on the amount of force required to flatten a specific area of the central cornea. Indentation tonometers, on the other hand, use a known force and measure the amount of resulting corneal indentation.
- Normal eye pressures are between 10 and 21 mmHg and vary throughout the day [2].

Goldmann Applanation Tonometer

The Goldmann applanation tonometer is the gold standard of IOP measurement and is typically integrated into a mounted slit lamp. Note that the device can produce inaccurate readings in patients who have abnormal corneas, such as edematous or scarred corneas.

Instructions [2]

- Insert a clean tonometer tip into the tonometer biprism holder.
- Instill a topical anesthetic eye drop and fluorescein dye into the eyes.
- Seat the patient properly at the slit lamp.
- Place the cobalt filter in front of the slit lamp to highlight the fluorescein dye.
- Using a low power magnification on the slit lamp focus a high-intensity, wide-angle, light beam on the tip of the tonometer.
- Instruct the patient to look at the examiner's ear opposite the eye being measured and to blink once to properly distribute the dye.
- Advance the biprism towards the patient until it lightly contacts the cornea. Two semicircles will become visible when contact is made (see Fig. 2.3).
- Slowly adjust the force knob so that the inner border of the two semicircles touch and record the corresponding pressure reading.

Fig. 2.3 Goldmann applanation tonometer attached to a slit lamp biomicroscope

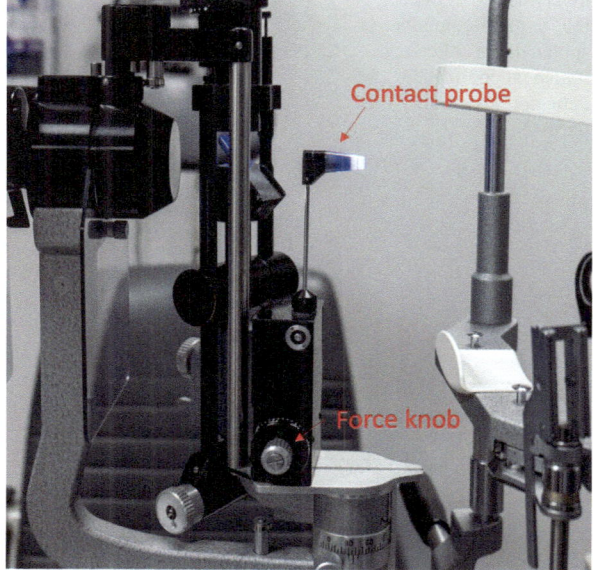

Common Handheld Tonometers

Tono-Pen [2]

The Tono-Pen is a handheld, electronic tonometer that utilizes a small plunger tip to measure the force needed to applanate the cornea (Fig. 2.4). It requires multiple readings, which are averaged to deliver the measured IOP.

- Calibrate the Tono-Pen at the beginning of each day.
- Instill a drop of topical anesthetic and placing a disposable sterile cover over the Tono-Pen tip. Depress the operator button to activate the device, ensure that no errors are reported on the device's screen.
- Ask the patient to look straight ahead with eyes open. Hold the Tono-Pen with a "pencil grip" and bring the probe tip in front of the patient's central cornea.
- Briefly and lightly touch the probe tip to the patient's eye, repeating until four valid readings are obtained and the average IOP measurement appears on the device's LCD display (device will also beep).
- Repeat for the fellow eye.

Fig. 2.4 Tono-pen XL with labeled parts. The activation button can also be used to select applanation mode. The LCD display shows the IOP in mmHg, number of applanations collected, statistical confidence indicator, and battery life status

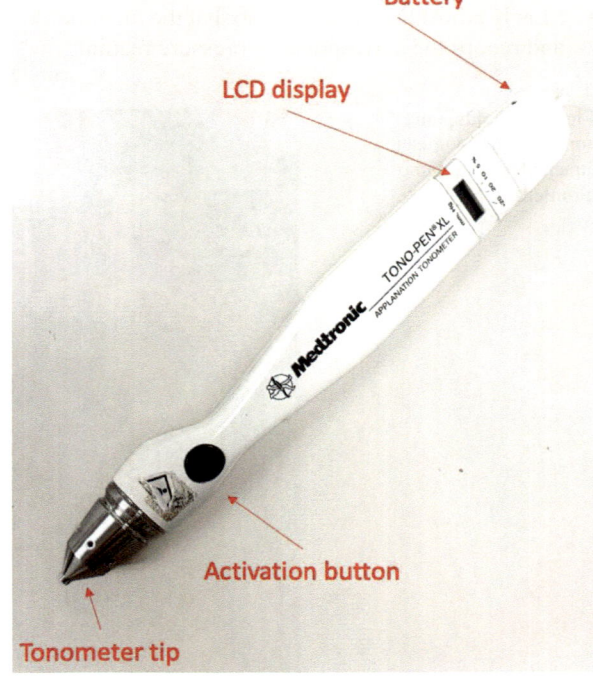

iCare Tonometer [2]

The iCare is another portable, handheld, tonometer in common use (Fig. 2.5). It utilizes a rebound mechanism to measure the IOP and takes the average of several measurements to deliver the final IOP. The primary advantage of this device is that it does not require topical anesthesia and is more convenient for pediatric and unco-operative patients.

- With the patient in a comfortable seated position ask the patient to look straight ahead with eyes open.
- Load the disposable sterile probe into the tonometer.
- Position and stabilize the iCare tonometer 4–8 mm away from the patient's eye.
- Press the measure button and repeat until 5 valid readings are recorded. The averaged IOP measurement will be displayed.
- Repeat for the fellow eye.

Fig. 2.5   iCare tonometer and parts labeled

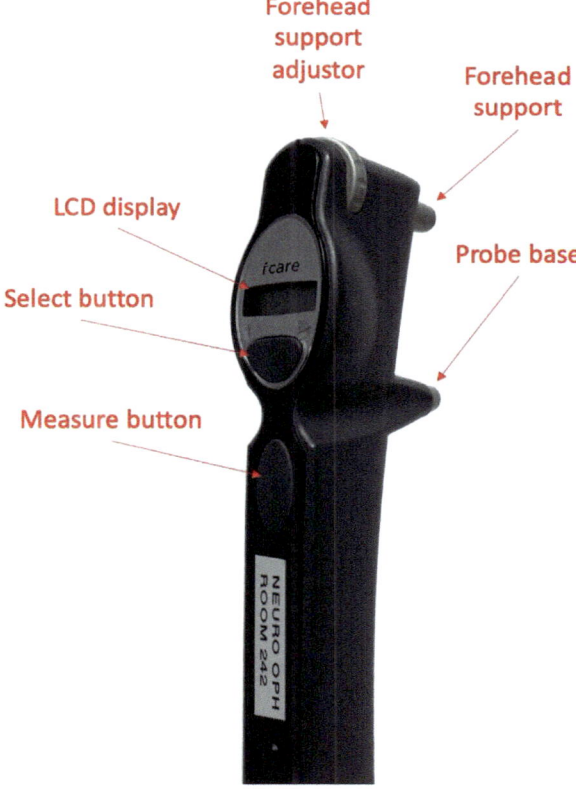

Perkins Tonometer

The Perkins tonometer relies on a similar mechanism to the Goldmann applanation tonometer, but it is a handheld device. Its portability comes at a cost of decreased accuracy as the stability of the device during measurements is not guaranteed.

Noncontact Tonometer

Noncontact tonometers measure the IOP by delivering a puff of air against the cornea and measuring the time it takes to flatten the central cornea. A noncontact tonometer is not recommended for patients with extremely high or low IOP.

Visual Field

A normal binocular visual field spans 170° along the horizontal meridian and 130° along the vertical meridian. Various methods test different ranges of the visual field. Characterization of visual field defects help make diagnoses, track progression of certain diseases over time, and assess patients' response to treatments.

Visual Field Testing

Confrontation Testing [1, 2]

- Seat the patient across from you and ask the patient to occlude one eye with his or her hand. As the examiner, close your eye that is directly across from the patient's occluded eye (your right eye if the patient has occluded his or her left eye).
- Compare your visual field to the patient's by moving an object, typically a single finger, in the periphery of each of the four quadrants. You can also ask the patient to count the number of fingers you have held up in the periphery. Record the differences in perception.

Amsler Grid [1, 2]

The Amsler grid is a handheld card that tests the central 20° of the visual field and is often used to evaluate macular function, especially when the patient experiences symptoms of central distortion/loss (Fig. 2.6). It is often given to patients to assess for macular edema at home.

Fig. 2.6 Amsler grid. It can also be commonly seen with white background and black lines

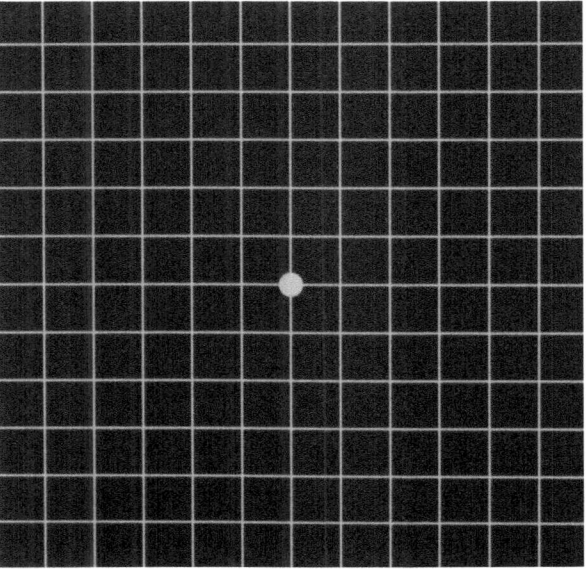

- Ask the patient to occlude their non-testing eye and hold out the testing grid appropriately 12 inches away. Ask the patient to focus on the central spot and assess whether any of part of the grid appears distorted or missing. Have the patient draw the distorted or missing parts. Repeat for the other eye.

Tangent Screen [1, 2]

Tangent screen test consists of a piece of black felt and a small white ball that measures the central 60° of vision (Fig. 2.7).

- Seat the patient 3–6 feet (1–2 m) away from the screen with one eye occluded. Move the small white ball centrally and record the location on the felt where the patient can first see the ball. Test blind spots with progressively larger objects to assess the severity of field loss.

Hemisphere Perimeters [1, 2]

A hemisphere perimeter is a machine that tests all degrees of the visual field and can be automated or manual (Fig. 2.8). Automated perimetry has the advantage of standardizing the visual stimulus and patient response but manual perimetry can still be used when patients are not able to operate the automated interface.

Fig. 2.7 Tangent screen
with blind spots marked

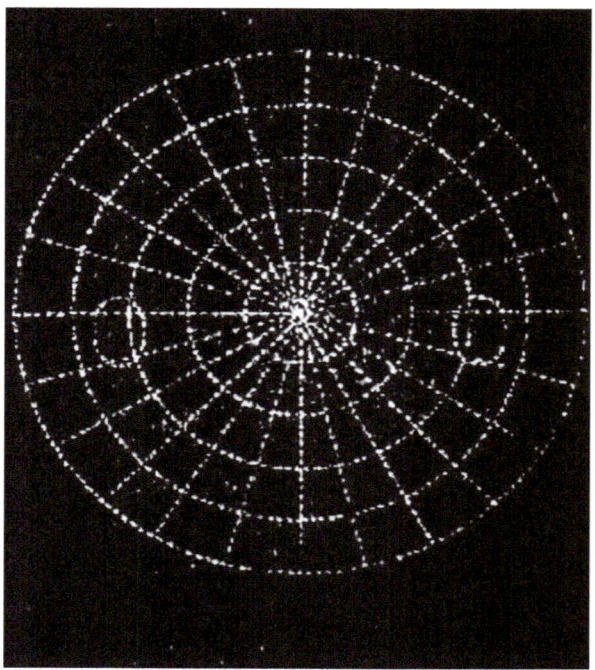

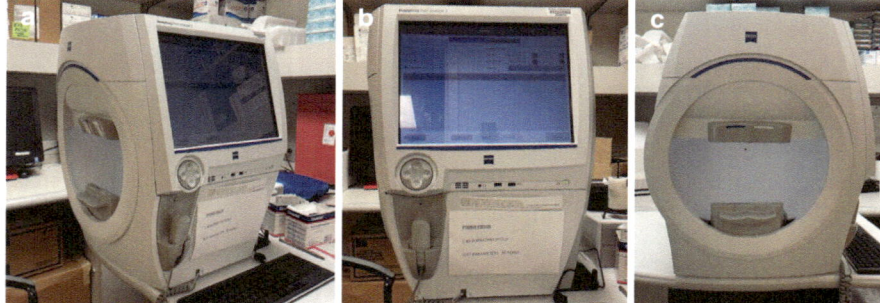

Fig. 2.8 (**a**) Side view of the Humphrey Field Analyzer (HFA). (**b**) Operator view of the HFA. (**c**) Patient view of the HFA

During automated testing, place the patient's head on the chinrest (Fig. 2.8c) and instruct them to fix their gaze towards the central point. Instruct the patient to trigger the machine (with handheld control) when they perceive a stimulus during testing. The examination tests various locations of the visual field until the threshold (the stimulus intensity seen 50% of the time) is determined at each location.

- The Swedish Interactive Threshold Algorithm (SITA) has become the preferred method for fast, reliable visual field testing. SITA has several testing protocols, including the 30–2, 24–2, and 10–2 program. The first number of the protocol

refers to the extent of visual field assessed in degrees from the center of fixation to the temporal side. The latter number refers to the version of the protocol.
- The 24–2 and 30–2 programs are used for general screening, early glaucoma, and neurological conditions.
- The 10–2 program is usually used for macular conditions or for conditions affecting predominantly the central visual field.

Anterior Segment

Slit-Lamp Examination (SLE) Introduction

The slit lamp microscope enables magnified (10–25 ×) stereoscopic examination of the anterior segment of the eye, including the eyelid, conjunctiva, cornea, anterior chamber, iris, posterior chamber, lens, and anterior vitreous cavity (Fig. 2.9). When used in conjunction with particular ophthalmic lenses, it also enables views to the anterior chamber angle and posterior segment. During the SLE, the patient is seated

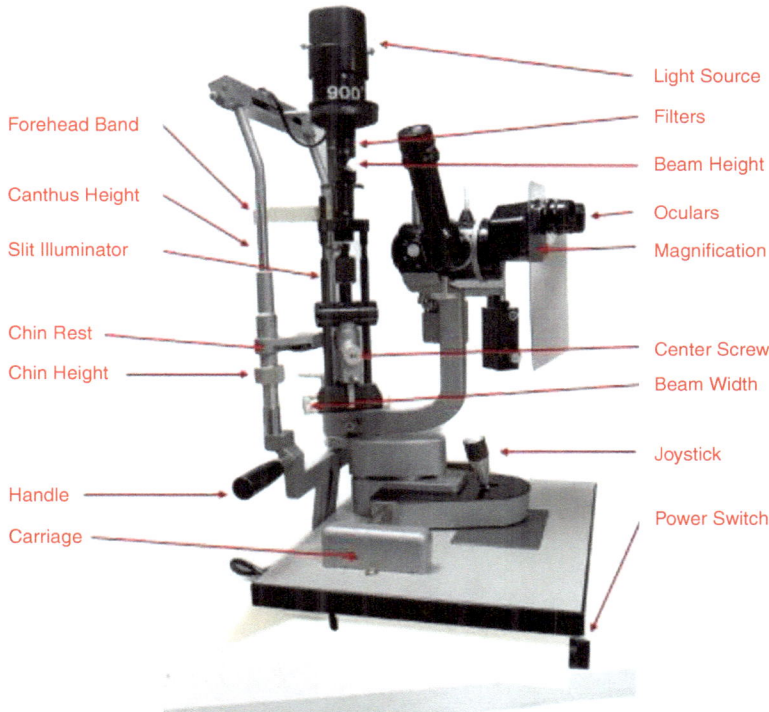

Fig. 2.9 Slit lamp biomicroscope with labeled components

with his or her head secured against a forehead strap and chin rest, while the examiner sits across from the patient looking through the binocular eyepiece. The slit lamp projects a beam of light of variable length, width, brightness, and color onto the patient's eye, enabling the examiner to scan surface structures, obtain cross-sectional views, and study cellular details [2, 3].

General Considerations

- There are no absolute contraindications for SLE, but caution should be taken for patients who cannot position at the lamp.
- The SLE is typically performed in a dimly-lit or completely dark setting.
- Examine the eyelids and eye in a methodical fashion. In general, advance from left to right, superiorly to inferiorly, and anteriorly to posteriorly. Begin with low magnification and diffuse lighting or direct focal illumination, then move to high magnification and more specialized illumination techniques as indicated.

Positioning [3]

- Adjust examiner chair height and inter-pupillary distance for comfort. Set ocular lenses to 0 diopters (examiner should wear their corrective lenses), and set the magnification to low power.
- Position patients in the chin rest and instruct them to keep their forehead in contact with the headrest at all times (Fig. 2.10). Adjust table height and chin rest such that the pupils are aligned with the horizontal marker.
- Focus the slit lamp by adjusting for a tall, narrow beam of white light directed on the bridge of the patient's nose. Use coarse focus to bring the slit into a crisp sharp focus as viewed externally. Then shift to using the eyepieces and use the fine focus joystick to obtain a crisp image under magnification.
- Confirm that the light beam is projected at a 45° angle in a temporal-to-nasal direction and move the assembly across the eye.

Fig. 2.10 Proper positioning of patient (left) and examiner (right) for a SLE

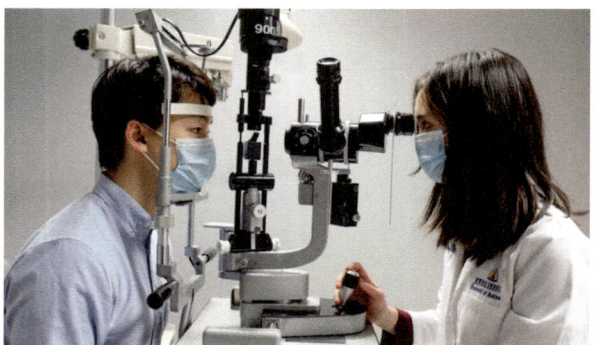

Eyelids and Conjunctiva [2, 3]

- Examine the upper and lower eyelids with focus on any skin lesions. Note the size, color, appearance, and location of each lesion. Assess for associated eyelash loss and distortion of normal eyelid anatomy.
- Evaluate the upper eyelid palpebral conjunctiva by everting the upper eyelid. Instruct the patient to look down and grasp the eyelashes while rolling the eyelid over a fulcrum (typically the wooden end of a cotton-tipped applicator) (Fig. 2.11a–d). Remove the applicator and hold the lid in everted position while panning the slit lamp horizontally across exposed palpebral conjunctiva.
- To evaluate the superior bulbar conjunctiva apply superior traction to the lid and ask the patient to look down. Move the slit beam from lateral to nasal to examine the entire bulbar conjunctiva. Examine for abrasions, swelling, or discharge using the slit lamp as necessary.

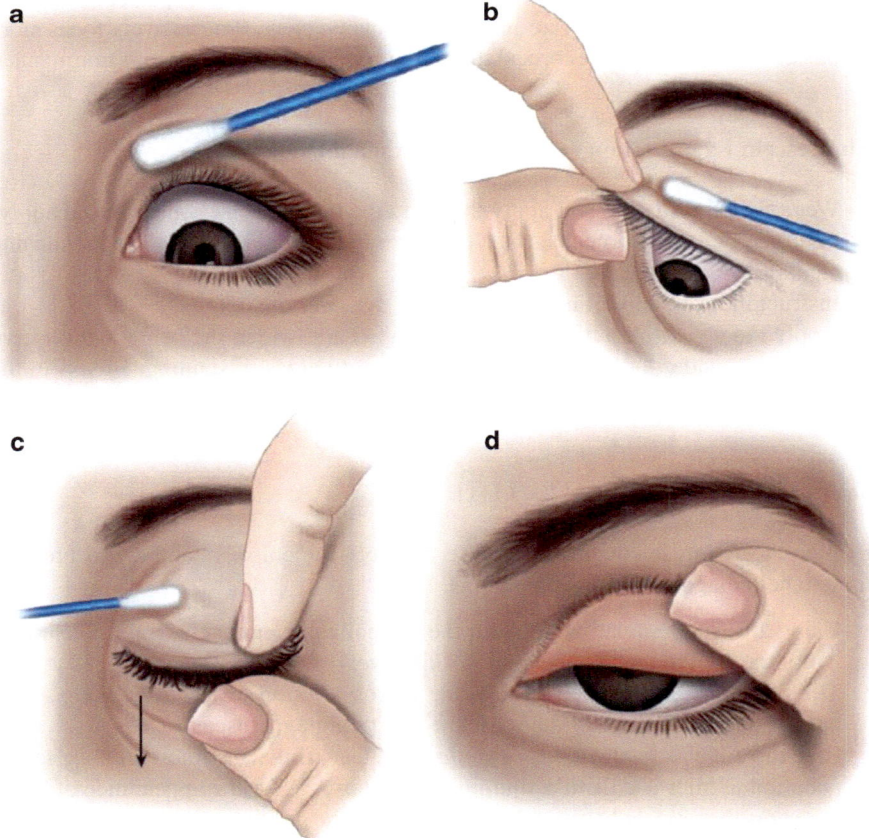

Fig. 2.11 (a–d) Procedure for everting the upper eyelid using a cotton-tipped applicator

- To evaluate the lower eyelid palpebral conjunctiva, instruct the patient to look up while the lower eyelid is manually pulled downward using a finger or cotton-tipped applicator. Pan slit lamp horizontally across exposed conjunctiva. The lower bulbar conjunctiva is then examined in a manner analogous to that used for the superior bulbar conjunctiva.
- The size of any lesions present can be measured by focusing a vertically oriented beam onto the lesion and adjusting the height of the beam until it equals the height of the lesion. The scale on the slit lamp indicates beam height (and thus lesion height) in 0.1 mm units. The beam can be rotated 90° and adjusted to measure the horizontal dimension.

Cornea [1]

- Focus the light beam on the nasal or temporal limbus at a 45° angle set on low magnification before sliding the assembly left and right horizontally to view the corneal epithelium. If abnormalities are present, switch to higher power to examine more closely and note the size and depth of involvement. Progressively focus more posteriorly to examine the corneal stromal and endothelial layers in the same manner.

Fluorescein Examination for Corneal Epithelial Defects [1]

- Wet a fluorescein strip and apply the tip to the lower fornix gently. Avoid applying directly to the corneal surface (except when Seidel testing) to avoid causing an abrasion.
- Instruct the patient to blink, spreading the dye over the cornea.
- Apply the cobalt blue filter to the slit lamp beam, widen the beam and observe the cornea under low and high power to identify areas of staining. Breaks in the cornea's epithelium fluoresce brightly under the cobalt blue filter.

Tear Film Breakup Time (TBUT) [1]

Evaluate tear film for quality (presence of debris), meniscus height, and breakup time to help diagnose dry eye syndrome.

- Using diffuse illumination, look for the normally glistening character of tear film in contrast to the matte appearance of dry eye.
- The meniscus is evaluated by viewing a cross-section of tear film using a tall, narrow beam, looking for the presence of a triangle meniscus.
- Breakup time is evaluated by staining the tear film with fluorescein. Use the cobalt blue filter and diffuse illumination to observe for the appearance of black dry spots that appear between blinks, counting the number of seconds that elapse between each blink and appearance of the first dry spot (normal is 10 s or greater).

Anterior Chamber [2, 3]

Under normal circumstances the anterior chamber should be transparent. The presence of opacities is indicative of pathology and may be observed at the slit lamp.

- To examine the anterior chamber adjust the light beam to an approximately 1 × 1 mm beam focused midway between cornea and iris.
- Examine the anterior chamber for "flare" (resembles smoke floating in beam of light) and cell (small, mobile, refractile points in the light beam). The presence of cell or flare is indicative of pathology.
- Instructing the patient to perform rapid saccades several times will agitate any floating opacities in the aqueous humor and make them more apparent.
- The slit lamp may also be used to approximate anterior chamber depth in the context of evaluating acute angle closure glaucoma risk. Prior to applying dilating drops to the eye, direct the slit beam towards the corneal periphery at an angle of 60° to observe the distance between the iris and inner surface of the cornea. A distance less than ¼ of the corneal thickness or evidence of peripheral contact between the iris root and cornea is indicative of increased risk for angle closure.

Iris [1, 3]

The surface of the iris and pupillary margin may be examined using direct illumination to examine for irregularities in pigmentation, lesions, asymmetry, or neovascularization.

- Transillumination may be used to detect abnormalities in the iris against a backlit retina. Adjust the light to a short, narrow beam and shine directly through the pupil. Observe the iris for any evidence of transmitted light reflected from the retina.

Lens [3]

- Using a narrow beam, an optical section of the lens reveals its multilaminar structure (capsule, cortex, and nucleus). The slit lamp is therefore an ideal tool for evaluating cataracts. Anterior capsular cataracts and nuclear sclerosis may be detected using direct illumination, while posterior capsular and subcapsular cataracts are best viewed with retroillumination.
- The slit lamp may also be used to evaluate the natural or prosthetic lens for dislocation (trauma or connective tissue disorders).

Posterior Segment

Examination of the posterior segment can be performed using a direct ophthalmo-scope, indirect ophthalmoscope, or slit lamp biomicroscope. This section will cover direct and indirect ophthalmoscopy.

Direct Ophthalmoscopy

Overview

- The direct ophthalmoscope is a handheld instrument that consists of a light source, viewing aperture, and a variety of built-in filters and openings to adjust light intensity and pattern (Fig. 2.12).
- The direct ophthalmoscope produces an erect, virtual image of the retina at 15 × magnification with a 5° field of view.
- Direct ophthalmoscopy is appropriate for examining the optic nerve head and associated blood vessels.

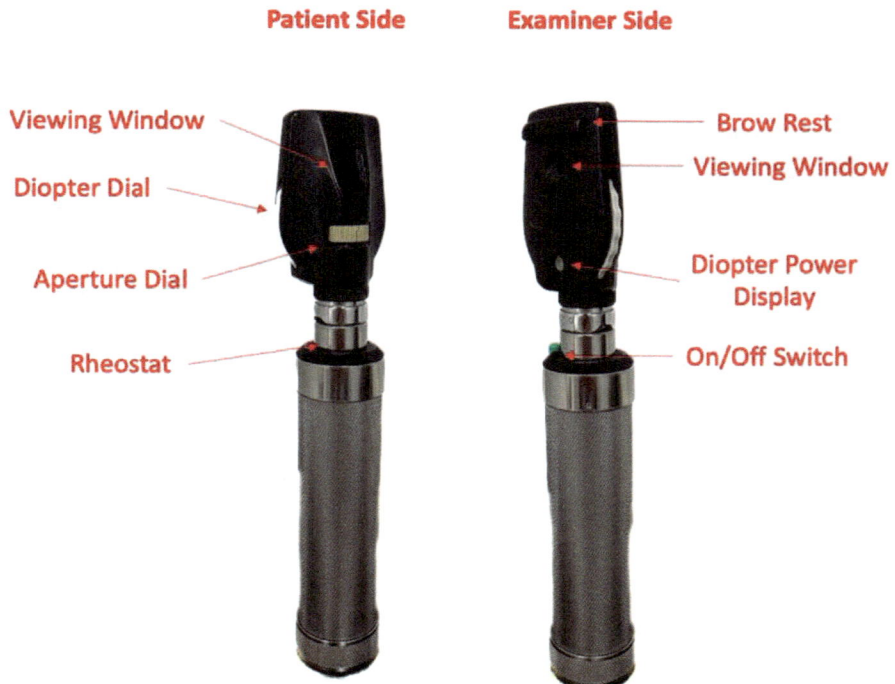

Fig. 2.12 Direct ophthalmoscope and parts labeled

Examination [1]

- At a distance of 2 feet (0.6 m) evaluate the patient's red reflex to assess for any opacities in the refractive media.
- Bring the eye that corresponds to the patient's eye (i.e., your left eye with the patient's left) to the viewing aperture of the ophthalmoscope.
- Adjust the focus of the ophthalmoscope using the dial on the back of the ophthalmoscope to focus on the iris to check for refractive media and vitreous floaters.
- Instruct the patient to look into the distance and adjust the focus to the fundus.
- Angle the ophthalmoscope approximately 15° temporally and center the light beam to properly visualize the optic disc and surrounding retina. A green filter can be used to enhance the visibility of the nerve fibers.

Indirect Ophthalmoscopy

Overview

- Indirect ophthalmoscopy allows for posterior segment evaluation and has the advantages of stereopsis, a large field of view, and the ability to incorporate scleral depression for far peripheral examination.
- An indirect ophthalmoscope consists of a binocular headset with a light source and a variety of ophthalmic lenses held between you and the patient's eye (Fig. 2.13). The image is stereoscopic, inverted, and reversed.

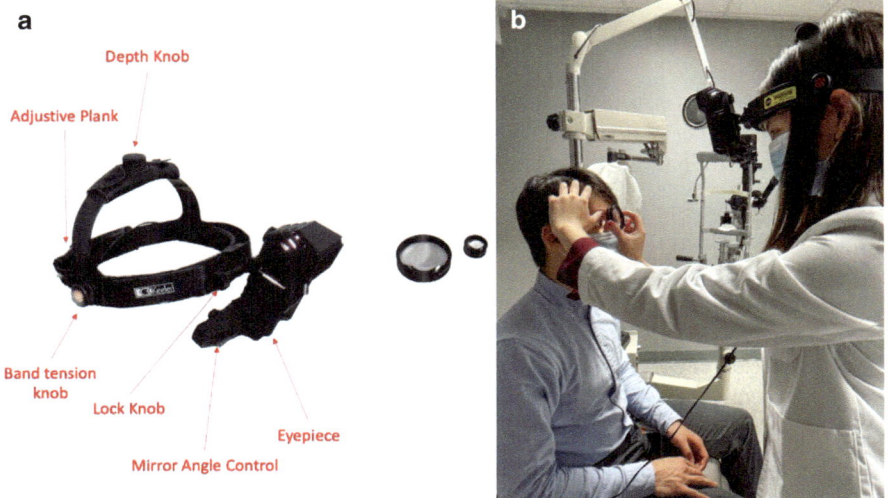

Fig. 2.13 (**a**) Indirect ophthalmoscope headset and viewing lens. (**b**) Examination of patient's right eye using indirect ophthalmoscope

- The image magnification varies based on the lens used during the exam. The +20 D lens is typically used for a routine eye examination. The +14 D lens provides higher magnification and can be used to examine the details of the optic disc with a smaller field of view, while the +30 D lens provides lower magnification for a wider view and is useful for smaller pupils.

Headset Adjustment

- Position the eyepiece close to your eyes without touching the bridge of your nose.
- Adjust the interpupillary distance so that you have a comfortable binocular view at arm's length.

Lens Position and Examination [2]

- Hold the appropriate lens between your thumb and index finger of your non-dominant hand with the convex side facing towards you. Use the middle finger of your non-dominant hand and the thumb of your dominant hand to keep the patient's eyelids open.
- Adjust the position of the lens so that the target area's image is entirely and uniformly filling the lens. You may also need to adjust the size and brightness of the light beam.
- Begin examination by identifying the optic disc and macula before moving to the periphery.

Scleral Depression [1, 2]

Scleral depression is a technique performed during indirect ophthalmoscopy to visualize the far peripheral retina and ora serrata. This examination is used to identify peripheral retinal breaks and chorioretinal lesions.

- Hold the depressor between your thumb, index, and middle fingers of your dominant hand. Depression can be applied directly on the globe (after instilling an anesthetic eyedrop) or through the eyelid.
- Gently apply pressure using the depressor, slide the depressor anteriorly, adjust the condensing lens if needed, and ask the patient to look in an extreme gaze in the direction of the depressor while you stand on the opposite side of the eye.
- Methodically repeat the process by moving clockwise or counterclockwise around the eye until you have examined the entire periphery.

References

1. Leitman MW. Manual for eye examination and diagnosis. New York: Wiley Blackwell; 2017.
2. American Academy of Ophthalmology. Practical ophthalmology: a manual for beginning residents. 6th ed. San Francisco: American Academy of Ophthalmology; 2009.
3. Knoop KJ. Slit-lamp examination. In: Post TW, editor. UpToDate. Waltham: UpToDate; 2022.

Chapter 3
Oculoplastics and Periocular Oncology

Hannah Miller, Rebecca Li, and Christopher J. Hwang

Anatomy

Orbit Anatomy [1, 2]

- The bony orbit consists of seven bones which protect and house the globe, extraocular muscles, arteries, nerves, and fat (Fig. 3.1). The average orbital volume is 30 mL. The **superior orbital fissure** divides the greater and lesser wings of the sphenoid and provides a path for nerves, arteries, and veins to enter the orbit. The optic nerve passes through the **optic canal** within the lesser wing of the sphenoid bone. Surrounding the central superior orbital fissure and optic canal is the fibrous **annulus of Zinn**, which is the origin for the four rectus muscles.
- Bones of the orbital roof:
    - frontal bone and lesser wing of the sphenoid bone
- Bones of the orbital floor:
    - maxillary, palatine, and zygomatic bones
    - frequently fractured in facial trauma (i.e., orbital blow out fracture)
- Bones of the lateral wall:
    - zygomatic and greater sphenoid bones
    - the lateral wall is the strongest wall of the orbit
- Bones of the medial wall:

H. Miller · R. Li · C. J. Hwang (✉)
Department of Ophthalmology, University of North Carolina at Chapel Hill, Chapel Hill, NC, USA
e-mail: Hannah.miller2@unchealth.unc.edu; Rebecca.li@unchealth.unc.edu; christopher_hwang@med.unc.edu

© The Author(s), under exclusive license to Springer Nature Switzerland AG 2023
E. Li, C. Bacorn (eds.), *Ophthalmology Clerkship*, Contemporary Surgical Clerkships, https://doi.org/10.1007/978-3-031-27327-8_3

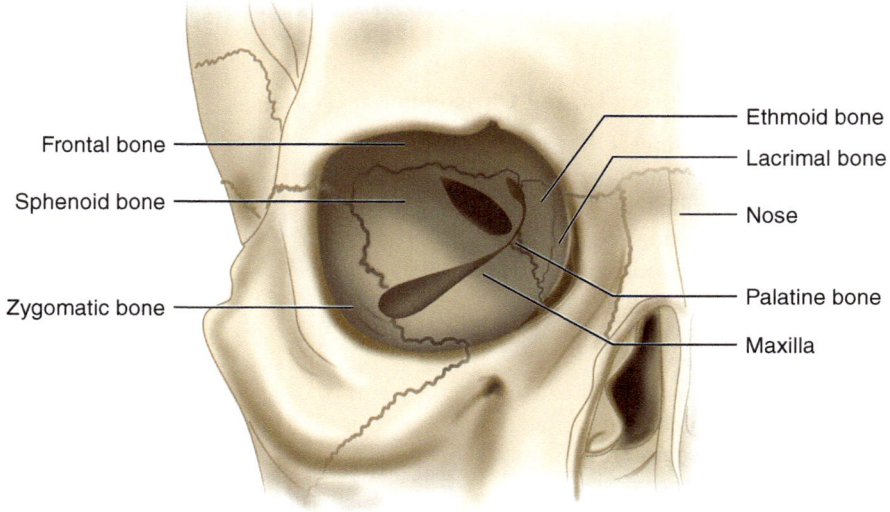

Fig. 3.1 Bones of the orbit

- ethmoid, lacrimal, maxillary, and lesser wing of the sphenoid

Eyelid Anatomy [1, 2]

- The eyelids protect the eye and maintain a lubricated ocular surface. The eyelids are composed of seven layers (Fig. 3.2):
  - skin and subcutaneous tissue
  - muscles of protraction (close the eye)
  - orbital septum
  - orbital fat
  - muscles of retraction (open the eye)
  - tarsus
  - palpebral conjunctiva
- The **tarsus** is composed of compact connective tissue and provides structural support to the eyelid. The tarsi are tapered at each end and attach to the periosteum of the orbital rim through the canthal tendons. These attachments determine the contour of the palpebral fissure and are essential for maintaining normal lid position.

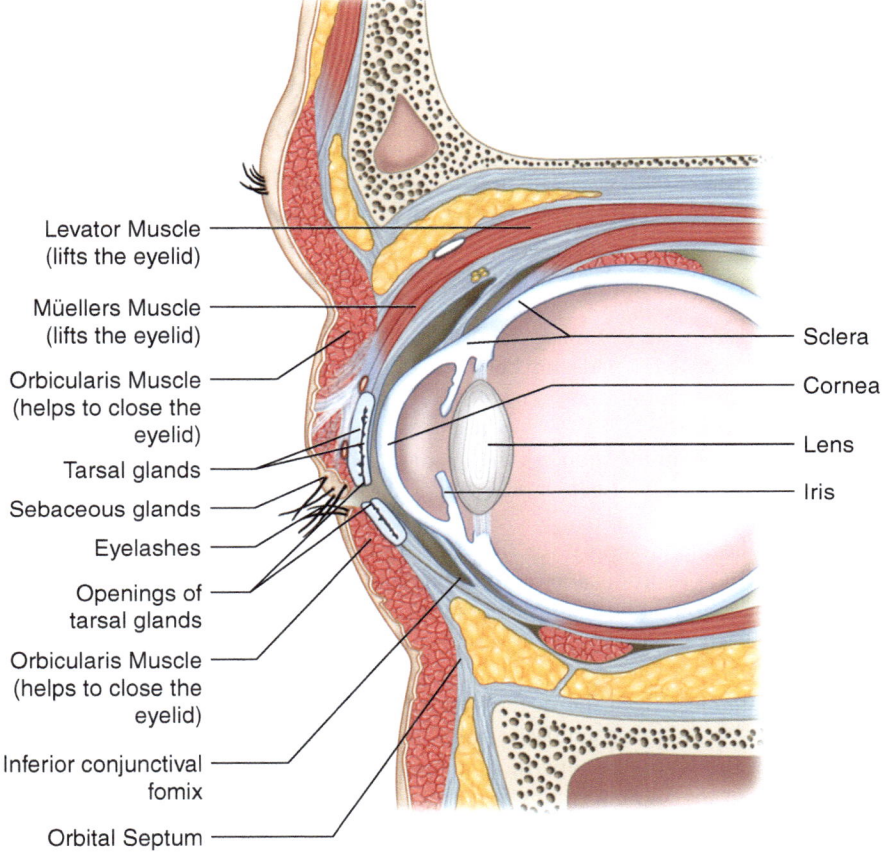

Fig. 3.2 Eyelid anatomy

- **Meibomian glands** are vertically oriented glands within the tarsus that contribute to the lipid layer of the tear film via openings along the eyelid margin.
- The **orbicularis oculi** is an annular muscle innervated by cranial nerve VII (CN VII) and is the primary protractor of the eyelid. The palpebral portion is responsible for involuntary eyelid movements (such as blinking). The orbital portion is responsible for voluntary eyelid closure. The gray line of the eyelid margin is formed by the pretarsal orbicularis muscle (also called the muscle of Riolan).
- The muscles of retraction for the upper eyelid are the **levator** palpebrae superioris and **Müller's muscle**. The levator originates from the lesser wing of the sphenoid and has a robust tendon/aponeurosis anteriorly which inserts along the anterior face of the tarsus. It is innervated by cranial nerve III (CN III). Müller's muscle originates from beneath the levator muscle and inserts on the superior

border of the tarsal plate. Müller's muscle is innervated by the sympathetic nervous system and provides approximately 2–3 mm of elevation for the upper eyelid.

- In the lower eyelid, the inferior tarsal muscle is analogous to Müller's muscle and capsulopalpebral fascia is analogous to the levator aponeurosis. These structures serve to retract the lower eyelid.
- The **orbital septum** is a thin, fibrous, sheet of tissue that arises from the periosteum of the orbital rim. The upper eyelid septum fuses with the levator aponeurosis and is an important barrier preventing the spread of infection into the orbit.
- There are two fat pads in the upper eyelid and three in the lower eyelid. In the upper eyelid, the central and medial fat pads lie posterior to the septum and anterior to the levator aponeurosis. In the lower eyelid, the medial, central, and lateral fat pads lie between the septum and the capsulopalpebral fascia. The medial and central fat pads are separated by the inferior oblique muscle.
- **Whitnall's ligament** supports the upper eyelid and functions as a fulcrum for the levator muscle. Lockwood's ligament is an analogous structure in the lower eyelid.
- The arterial blood supply for the eyelids comes from the internal (ICA) and external (ECA) carotid arteries (via ophthalmic, facial, and angular branches) which the marginal and peripheral arcades. These arcades allow form a watershed between the ICA and ECA and provide robust blood flow to the eyelid structures.
- Venous drainage from the eyelid can be divided into preseptal and postseptal drainage. Medial preseptal tissue drains into the angular vein and lateral preseptal tissues drain into the superficial temporal vein. Venous blood from structures posterior to the septum drains into the anterior facial vein, orbital veins, and pterygoid plexus.
- The lymphatic vessels of the medial eyelid drain into submandibular lymph nodes and lateral lymphatic vessels drain into superficial preauricular lymph nodes.

Lacrimal System Anatomy [3]

- The lacrimal system can be divided into secretory (tear producing) and excretory (tear draining) systems.
- The **lacrimal gland** is the primary tear-producing exocrine gland and is located in the superior lateral orbit. The gland is divided into orbital and palpebral lobes by the levator aponeurosis.
- Accessory lacrimal glands, the Glands of Krause and Wolfring, are located within the conjunctival fornices and along the superior tarsal border, respectively, and also contribute to tear production.

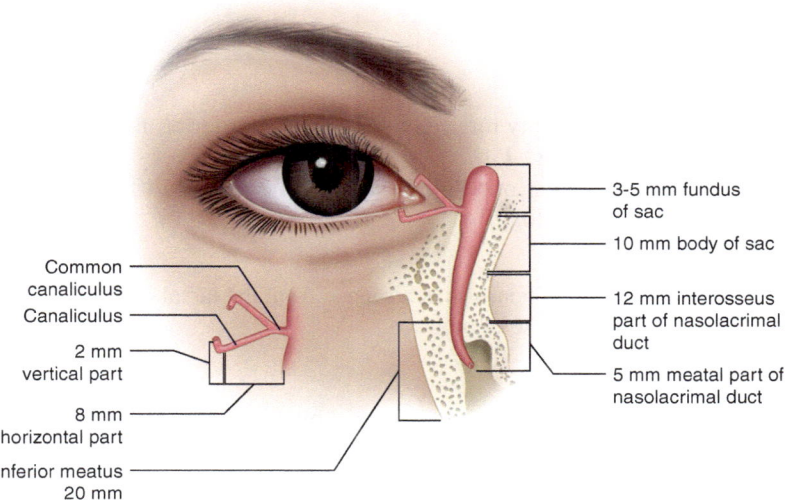

Fig. 3.3 Excretory lacrimal system

Fig. 3.4 Ptosis

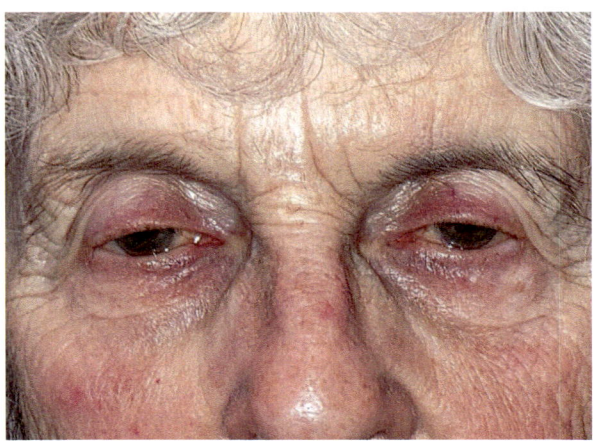

- The excretory portion of the lacrimal system begins with the **puncta**, which are small openings in the medial eyelid margins (Fig. 3.3). The punctum of each lid drains into a **canaliculus**. The upper and lower canaliculi join to form the common canaliculus, which drains into the lacrimal sac. Finally, tears drain from the lacrimal sac through the **nasolacrimal duct** into the inferior meatus of the nose.

Ptosis [3]

Blepharoptosis

- Blepharoptosis, commonly referred to as **ptosis**, is inferior displacement of the upper eyelid margin (Fig. 3.4).
- Ptosis can be congenital or acquired and can be further differentiated by the underlying pathophysiology:
  - Aponeurotic

    Due to levator aponeurosis dehiscence from the tarsal plate
    Most common cause of ptosis

  - Myogenic

    Congenital myogenic ptosis is caused by dysgenesis of the levator muscle resulting in decreased function
    Acquired myogenic ptosis occurs secondary to a muscular disease such as myotonic dystrophy, oculopharyngeal dystrophy, chronic progressive external ophthalmoplegia, or myasthenia gravis (MG)

  - Neurogenic

    Horner syndrome, CN III palsy, myasthenia gravis, Marcus Gunn jaw-winking syndrome
  - Mechanical

    Mass lesions (tumors, edema) depressing the eyelid
    Scar tissue tethering the eyelid in a ptotic position

  - Traumatic

    Surgical trauma, blunt force trauma, lacerations may all mechanically disrupt eyelid function

Ptosis Evaluation [3]

- The first step of any ptosis evaluation is to obtain a detailed history from the patient including length of symptoms, history of trauma or recent surgeries, systemic symptoms, and variability of ptosis.
- Examine brow position, facial symmetry, lid position, presence of excess skin on the eyelid (**dermatochalasis**), pupil reaction, and extraocular movements (Fig. 3.5).
- Evaluation involves several key measurements:

  - Margin-reflex distance (MRD)—distance from corneal light reflex to lid margin (MRD1) (Fig. 3.6).

    MRD2 is the distance from the lower eyelid margin to the corneal light reflex.

Fig. 3.5 Dermatochalasis (note excess upper eyelid skin over hanging lashes)

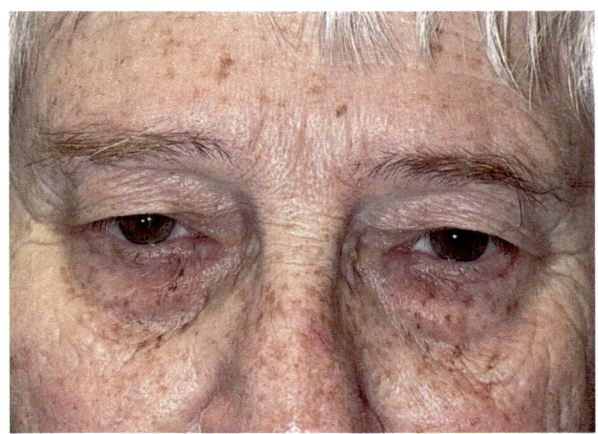

Fig. 3.6 Eyelid measurements (*MRD* margin-reflex distance, *PFH* palpebral fissure height). (Source: https://www.ophthalmologyreview.org/bcsc-fundamentals/eyelid-anatomy)

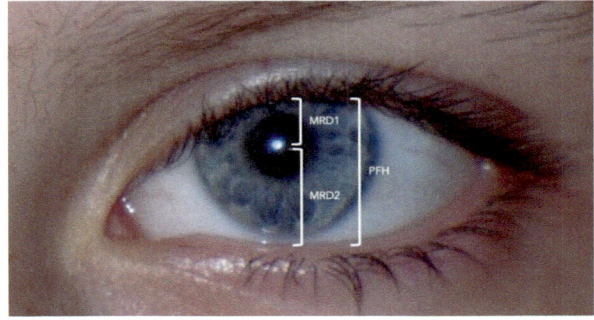

- Vertical palpebral fissure (PF) height—distance from the upper lid margin to the lower lid margin.
- Upper eyelid crease position—distance from lid margin to central lid crease.

    Absent or abnormally high (>10 mm) upper eyelid crease may indicate aponeurotic ptosis.

- Levator function—magnitude of eyelid margin excursion from down gaze to up gaze with the frontalis muscle fixated.
- Lagophthalmos—vertical distance between eyelid margins when closed.
- Additional work up may be warranted in specific cases of ptosis:

    - Horner's syndrome and CN III palsy—neuroimaging to evaluate for aneurysm or intracranial lesions.
    - Myasthenia gravis—Assess for fatigability on exam, double vision, difficulty swallowing, or axial muscle weakness. Additional testing may include ice-pack test, CT of the chest, and lab work evaluating for autoantibodies.

Ptosis Repair [3, 4]

- There are three main techniques for surgical repair of ptosis:
  - External levator advancement (ELA).
  - Müller's muscle-conjunctival resection (MMCR).
  - Frontalis muscle suspension.
- ELA is often performed in cases of levator dehiscence/aponeurotic ptosis. In this technique an incision is made at the upper eyelid crease and the tarsus and levator tendon are isolated. The levator aponeurosis is then advanced and secured to tarsal plate.
- The MMCR involves a graded transconjunctival resection of Müller's muscle and conjunctiva followed by advancement of these tissues to the superior border of the tarsus [4].
- If a patient has poor (<4 mm of excursion) or absent levator function, a frontalis muscle suspension may be indicated to correct the ptosis. In this procedure, the upper eyelid is suspended from the frontalis muscle using autogenous, allogenic, or synthetic material; and elevation of the brow is required to raise the eyelid.

Lower Eyelid Malposition [3]

Ectropion

- **Ectropion** is characterized by outward rotation of the lower eyelid margin away from the surface of the eye. There are five primary types of ectropion: congenital, cicatricial, paralytic, mechanical, and involutional (Fig. 3.7).
- Congenital ectropion is often associated with a genetic syndrome and is caused by insufficiency of the anterior lamella.
- Cicatricial ectropion results from scarring of the eyelid skin and can occur secondary to chemical or thermal burns, actinic damage, trauma, or inflammatory skin conditions.
- Paralytic lower eyelid ectropion occurs in cases of CN VII palsy. It is typically associated with poor lid closure and can lead to exposure keratopathy.
- Mechanical ectropion usually develops secondary to a lesion of the lower eyelid.
- Involutional ectropion is primarily due to horizontal lid laxity and inadequate attachments to the orbital rim. This form of ectropion is typically seen in older patients.
- Surgical correction of ectropion is tailored toward the underlying pathophysiology. Horizontal laxity may be addressed with a lateral tarsal strip (LTS) which shortens the eyelid and strengthens the lids attachment to the lateral orbital rim. Cicatricial ectropion often requires skin grafting to correct eyelid position.

Fig. 3.7 Ectropion

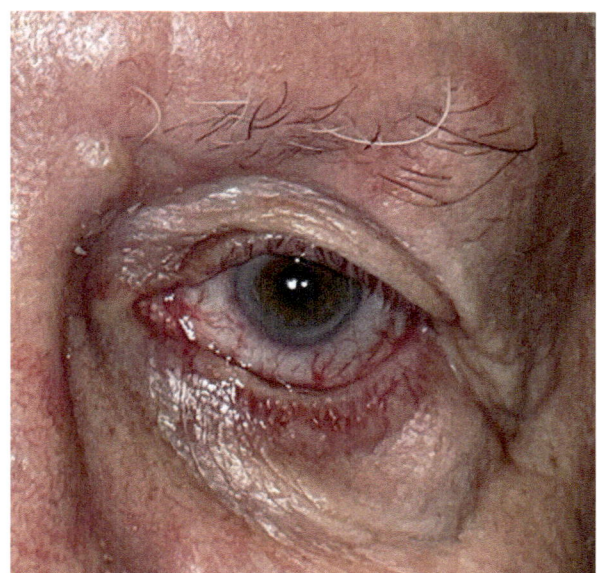

Fig. 3.8 Lower lid entropion

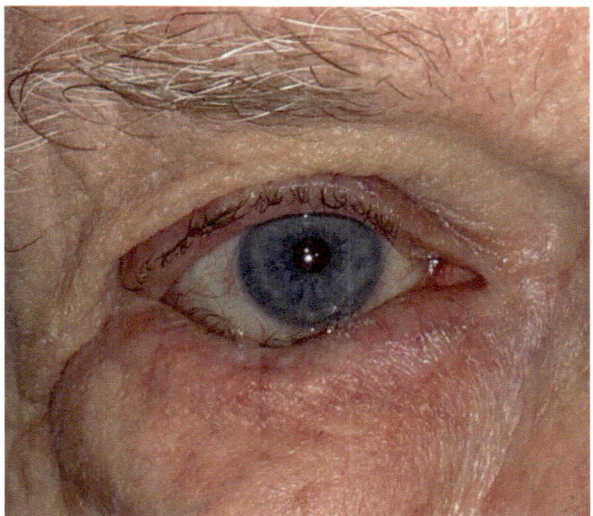

Entropion

- **Entropion** is characterized by inward rotation of the lower eyelid margin toward the eye. Like ectropion, there are congenital, involutional, and cicatricial causes of entropion (Fig. 3.8).
- Entropion can be caused by overaction of orbicularis muscle, often in the setting of lower eyelid laxity, and is referred to as acute spastic entropion.

- Congenital entropion is rare and is a result of developmental abnormalities of the tarsal plate.
- Involutional entropion occurs secondary to eyelid laxity and disinsertion or weakening of the eyelid retractors.
- Cicatricial entropion results from scarring and contraction of the palpebral conjunctiva. Ocular cicatricial pemphigoid, chronic conjunctivitis, and Steven Johnson Syndrome are all known causes of entropion. Upper eyelid entropion can also occur in the setting of trachoma and result in upper eyelid trichiasis and ocular surface scarring.
- Entropion repair generally involves some combination of reattaching the lower eyelid retractors to the tarsus, resection of the overriding orbicularis, and horizontally tightening the lower eyelid. Cicatricial entropion repair often requires grafting of the posterior lamella (for instance, from the mucus membranes of the mouth).

Eyelid Lesions [3, 5, 6]

Evaluation of Periocular Neoplasms

- Benign and malignant neoplasms can arise from the eyelid structures. When evaluating eyelid lesions, it is important to obtain a detailed history about the lesion and the patient's risk factors. Patient history should include:
  - History of sun exposure/sunburns
  - History of precancerous or cancerous lesions
  - Prior radiation treatment
  - Smoking history
  - History of immunocompromise (HIV/AIDS, cancers, or immunosuppressive medications)
  - Duration of lesion
  - Changes in appearance/size
  - Presence or absence of pain and bleeding
- There are several signs that may point to malignancy including:
  - Ulceration
  - Bleeding/non-healing lesion
  - Loss of normal eyelid structures such as hair follicles (**madarosis**), meibomian glands, and eyelid margin architecture
  - Pigmentary changes
  - Prominent blood vessels (telangiectasias)

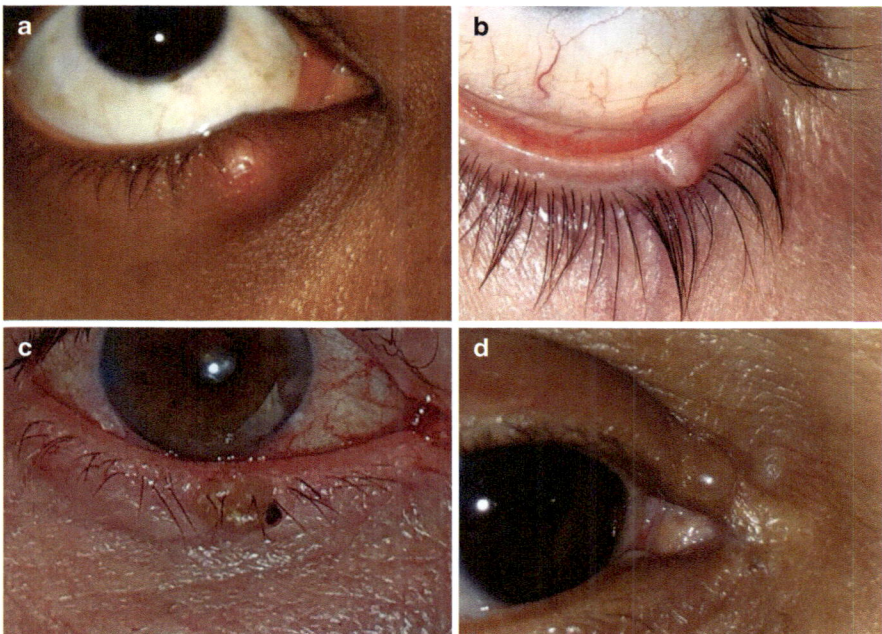

Fig. 3.9 Benign eyelid lesions; (**a**) Chalazion, (**b**) dermal nevus, (**c**) seborrheic keratosis, (**d**) hidrocystoma

Benign Lesions of the Eyelid

- Lesions arising from the periocular epithelial tissue are the most common benign eyelid lesions. Common epithelial lesions include papillomas, seborrheic keratosis, skin tags, xanthelasmas, molluscum contagiosum, and epidermal inclusion cysts (Fig. 3.9a–d).
- Benign lesions may arise from other structures within the eyelid such as the sebaceous oil glands, eyelash follicles, and eccrine sweat glands.
- **Chalazia** and **hordeola** (styes) are inflammatory lesions resulting from blockage of the sebaceous oil glands. Conservative treatment involves regular warm compresses and topical antibiotic or anti-inflammatory medications. If conservative measures fail surgical excision may be required.
- Neoplasms originating from the eccrine sweat glands include eccrine hidrocystomas, syringomas, and pleomorphic adenomas.
- Tumors arising from the hair follicles include trichoepithelioma, trichofolliculoma, trichilemmoma, and pilomatricoma.
- Benign melanocytic skin lesions commonly seen in the periocular region include nevi, ephelides (freckles), lentigo simplex, dermal melanocytosis, melasma, and blue nevi.

Fig. 3.10 Basal cell carcinoma

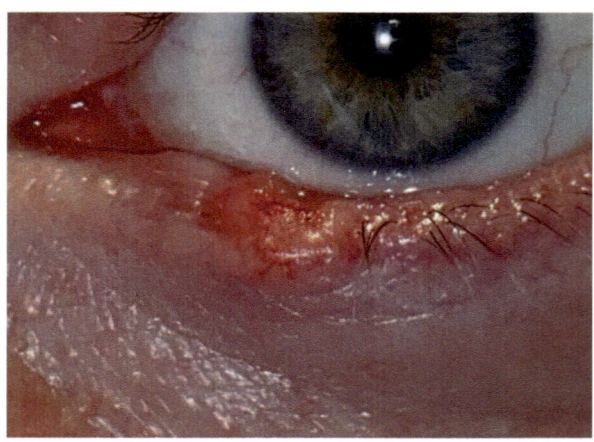

Malignant Lesions of the Eyelid [3, 5, 6]

- **Basal cell carcinoma** (BCC) is the most common malignancy of the eyelid.

  - Risk factors for basal cell carcinoma include fair skin, sun exposure, and smoking.
  - Nodular basal cell carcinoma typically presents as a pearly, raised, lesion with ulceration and telangiectasia (Fig. 3.10). The morpheaform type of basal cell carcinoma is more aggressive and is more diffuse with indeterminate edges. Basal cell carcinoma may also present as chronic eyelid inflammation with madarosis.
  - Metastasis is uncommon in BCC.
  - Management of BCC starts with documentation of size, location, and characteristics of the lesion. Photographs of the lesion should be taken prior to biopsy, which is required to confirm the diagnosis.
  - After the diagnosis is confirmed Mohs micrographic surgery is the preferred method of excision to ensure clear margins and to conserve unaffected tissue.

- **Squamous cell carcinoma** (SCC) of the eyelid typically arises from areas of sun damaged skin or from a premalignant lesion (actinic keratosis).

  - Squamous cell carcinomas behave more aggressively than basal cell carcinomas and are more likely to metastasize.
  - Patients with a history of immunodeficiency or organ transplant are at higher risk.
  - Lesions are typically flat and scaly in appearance.
  - As for BCC Mohs surgery is the preferred treatment for SCC of the eyelid.

- **Sebaceous carcinoma** is an aggressive malignant lesion arising from meibomian glands, glands of Zeiss, or sebaceous glands.

  - Tumors often masquerade as benign lesions delaying diagnosis. Often, sebaceous carcinoma initially resembles chronic blepharitis or a chalazion.
  - Can be associated with gastrointestinal malignancy (Muir-Torre Syndrome).

- Full-thickness biopsy through the tarsal plate is needed to confirm the diagnosis of sebaceous carcinoma. Sebaceous carcinoma may exhibit pagetoid spread and map biopsies may be used to assess for satellite lesions in the surrounding conjunctiva.
- Wide local excision and even exenteration may be necessary for large tumors invading the orbit.

- Cutaneous **melanoma** may develop spontaneously from a melanocytic nevus or from a precancerous lesion known as lentigo maligna.
- Melanoma of the eyelid typically presents as a flat lesion with variable pigmentation and irregular borders. Lesions may ulcerate or bleed.
- The four forms of cutaneous melanoma are lentigo maligna melanoma, nodular, superficial spreading and acrolentiginous.
- Lentigo maligna melanoma is the most common form of head and neck melanoma and typically invades vertically.
- Cutaneous melanoma must be managed aggressively with wide excisions and confirmation that the margins are clear. Additional treatment with immunotherapy and checkpoint inhibitors may be indicated. Regional lymph node dissection may also be indicated.

Epiphora [3]

Overview

- **Epiphora** refers to overflow tearing due to an imbalance in tear production and tear outflow. True epiphora occurs in the setting of tear outflow obstruction.
- The most common lacrimal system abnormality is congenital nasolacrimal duct obstruction (NLDO).

  - Congenital NLDO is typically caused by blockage of the valve of Hasner at the distal nasolacrimal duct (NLD).
  - In the absence of acute infection (**dacryocystitis**), patients are treated conservatively with massage of the lacrimal sac (Crigler massage) and prophylactic topical antibiotics.
  - Majority of cases resolve without intervention in the first year of life. If symptoms persist, or if dacryocystitis develops, probing and placement of lacrimal duct stents is usually performed.

Evaluation

- When evaluating patients for tearing, the first step is obtaining a thorough history. Important history to obtain:

- – Determine whether tearing is constant or intermittent and whether tears are clear or mucoid or bloody.
- – Prior dacryocystitis.
- – Seasonal allergies or nasal congestion.
- – Prior midface trauma or surgeries.
- – Chemotherapy or radioactive iodine.

- It is important to differentiate pseudoepiphora from true epiphora. Pseudoepiphora is tearing in the absence of outflow obstruction and may be caused by ocular surface disease, lid malposition, infection, or trichiasis.
- The puncta should be evaluated for stenosis or occlusion. Compression of the lacrimal sac should be performed to elicit mucoid reflux which could indicate NLDO. If the patient notes a history of bloody tears or blood refluxes from the lacrimal sac, this should raise suspicion for malignancy.
- The dye disappearance test measures the time required for clearance of fluorescein dye from the tear film and assess the flow of tears through the lacrimal system. Manual irrigation may also be used to assess the patency of the lacrimal system.

Management

- Treat ocular surface disease/dry eye syndrome to eliminate overproduction component of epiphora.
- Eyelid malposition should also be addressed via surgical tightening and/or repositioning.
- Surgical management of acquired epiphora depends on the degree and location of outflow obstruction.

   - – Stenosis of the puncta may be addressed by enlargement of the puncta via dilation or snip punctoplasty.
   - – Canaliculoplasty can be performed for canalicular stenosis or obstruction. If canaliculoplasty cannot be performed, then a conjunctivodacryocystorhinostomy (cDCR) with insertion of a Jones tube may be required.

- Partial stenosis of the NLD may respond well to probing and stent placement, sometimes in conjunction with balloon dacryoplasty.
- Complete NLDO requires surgical repair with a **dacryocystorhinostomy** (DCR). In this procedure, a fistula is created between the lacrimal sac and the middle meatus of the nose which reestablishes passage of tears into the nose.

Trauma

Eyelid and orbital injuries span the spectrum of mechanisms from blunt force injuries to sharp penetrating injuries. Careful examination of the periocular region, eyelids, eye, and orbit is critical.

Eyelid Lacerations

- The examination of an eyelid laceration should involve assessment of the structures involved, the extent of the injury, and for the presence of any foreign bodies.
- A complete eye exam should accompany any periocular injury to assess for an associated open globe injury.
- Exposure orbital fat indicates violation of the orbital septum and potential deeper orbital involvement.
- Superficial skin lacerations can be sutured or allowed to granulate; topical antibiotic ointment should be applied to the skin following repair.
- Lacerations involving the lid margin require methodical reapproximating of the anterior and posterior lamellae to prevent notching or misalignment of the lid margin.
- Lacerations involving the canalicular system should be confirmed via punctal dilation and canalicular probing. Canalicular involving lacerations require repair with placement of a silicone stent to reduce the risk of canalicular obstruction and chronic epiphora.

Orbital Fractures [7]

- Orbital fractures are common in periorbital or facial trauma. A complete eye exam should accompany any injury with enough force to cause orbital fracture to rule out globe injury.
- Many orbital fractures may not require surgical repair and can be observed.
- Common indications for fracture repair include:

  - Extraocular muscle entrapment (pediatric trapdoor fractures)
  - Diplopia within 15° of primary gaze
  - Fracture of greater than 50% of the floor
  - Significant (>2 mm) enophthalmos or hypoglobus

Thyroid Eye Disease [8–10]

Overview

- Thyroid eye disease (TED), also known as Graves ophthalmopathy, is an inflammatory condition that affects the periocular and orbital tissues and is most commonly associated with Graves' disease. TED can also occur in patients with Hashimoto's thyroiditis and in patients with normal thyroid function.
- TED is caused by circulating immunoglobulins activating thyroid-stimulating hormone receptors (TSHR) and insulin-like growth factor I receptors (IGF-IR) in orbital fibroblasts. Fibroblast activation results in expansion and fibrosis of orbital tissues.
- Patients present with a wide spectrum of disease ranging from mild dry eye to marked **proptosis** and compressive optic neuropathy. Proptosis and eyelid retraction (unilateral or bilateral) are the most common presenting signs of TED.
- Severity of TED does not correlate with thyroid hormones (TSH, T3, T4).
- TED is six times more common in females than in males.
- Smoking is a major modifiable risk factor in developing TED and all patients should be counselled on smoke avoidance and cessation.

Diagnosis

- Diagnosis of TED is made based on characteristic clinical findings:
  - Eyelid retraction
  - Lid lag on downgaze
  - Eyelid edema and/or erythema
  - Chemosis or caruncle inflammation
  - Proptosis
  - Restricted eye movements
  - Compressive optic neuropathy

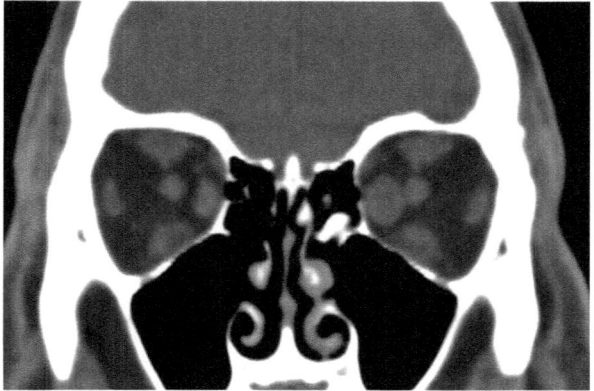

Fig. 3.11 Computed tomography demonstrating extraocular muscle enlargement from thyroid eye disease

- A history of auto-immune thyroid dysfunction is supportive, but TED can occur in the absence of thyroid dysfunction
  - Graves' disease—90%
  - Euthyroid—6%
  - Hashimoto thyroiditis—3%
  - Primary hypothyroidism—1%
- Laboratory studies can support the diagnosis of TED but are insufficient alone
  - Thyroid-stimulating hormone receptor (TSHR) antibodies, thyroid-stimulating immunoglobulins (TSI), anti-thyroid peroxidase antibody
- Radiographic evidence of TED
  - Enlargement of extraocular muscles (most frequently the inferior and medial recti) with sparing of the tendons (Fig. 3.11)
  - Orbital fat expansion may also be present
- The Clinical Activity Score (CAS) is frequently used to assess for active inflammation with 1 point given for each of the clinical signs below. A score of 3 or higher indicates active disease:
  - Spontaneous orbital pain
  - Gaze evoked orbital pain
  - Eyelid swelling due to TED
  - Eyelid erythema
  - Conjunctival redness due to TED
  - Chemosis
  - Inflammation of caruncle or plica

Management

Treatment of TED is dependent on the activity and severity of the disease:

- All disease: Smoking cessation
- Mild disease: Ocular lubricants, selenium supplementation
- Moderate disease: Topical cyclosporine, taping eyelids shut at night, moisture chambers, prism glasses or selective eye patching, oral corticosteroids
- Severe disease: High-dose steroids, orbital radiotherapy, surgical orbital decompression
- Teprotumumab: FDA-approved monoclonal antibody that inhibits IGF-IR activation and signaling, decreasing signs and symptoms of TED during active disease [11].
- Surgery to address proptosis, diplopia, or lid malposition can be performed in cases of inactive TED with stable exam findings.

Fig. 3.12 Periocular
edema and erythema in
orbital cellulitis

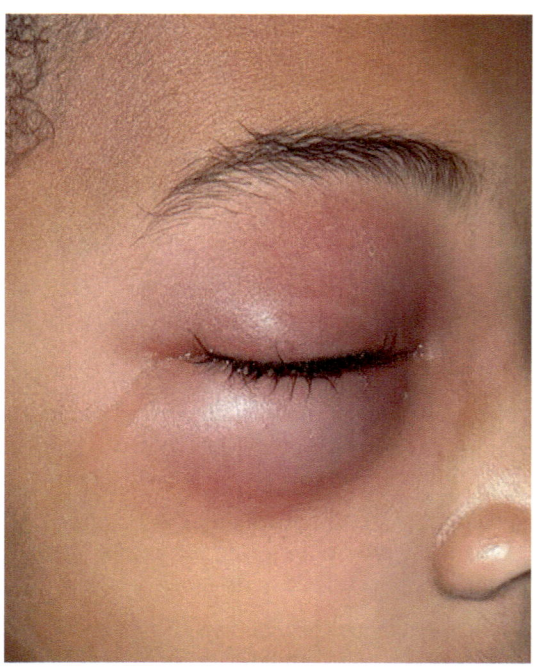

Fig. 3.13 Computed
tomography demonstrating
bilateral orbital abscesses

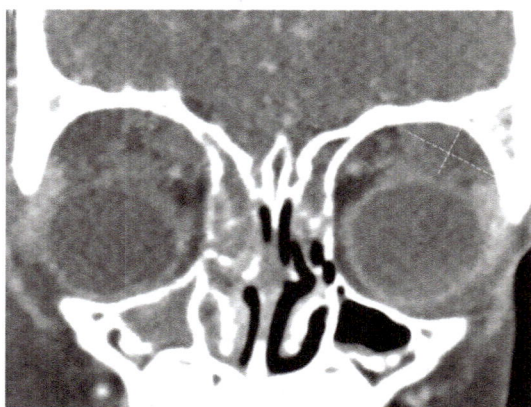

Orbital Infections

- **Preseptal cellulitis** is typically caused by a bacterial infection with streptococcal or staphylococcal species and occurs in tissues anterior to the orbital septum.
- **Orbital cellulitis** occurs when infection occurs in tissues that are posterior to the septum.
- Patients with periorbital infections typically present with acute periorbital edema and erythema (Fig. 3.12). When evaluating a patient obtain a history of any

recent infections, (especially sinus and odontogenic infections) periocular bug bites, or injuries.
- An exam should be performed to assess for orbital signs including:

  - afferent pupillary defect
  - decreased visual acuity
  - decreased color vision
  - visual field restriction
  - extraocular muscle restriction
  - proptosis

Management

- Preseptal cellulitis typically resolves with oral antibiotic therapy. Patients may require admission for intravenous antibiotics after failure of outpatient antibiotic course.
- Abscesses of the eyelid or orbit generally require incision and drainage.
- Orbital cellulitis requires hospitalization for intravenous antibiotics and CT imaging (Fig. 3.13).
  - Depending on the location and source of infection, collaboration with otolaryngology or dentistry to treat the source of infection may be required. If a subperiosteal abscess is present, surgical drainage may be indicated.

Eye Removal

- In some cases, such as a blind and painful eye, trauma, or malignancy, removal of the eye and/or orbital contents is indicated.
- Implants are often placed to maintain orbital volume and to allow for the wear of prostheses.
- Depending on the amount of tissue to be removed there are three general methods to remove the eye.

  - **Evisceration**: Removal of intraocular contents while sparing the sclera and extraocular muscles.
  - **Enucleation**: Removal of the entire globe, including the intact sclera, sparing the extraocular muscles.
  - **Exenteration**: Resection of the orbital contents including globe, extraocular muscles, and connective tissues. The eyelids may be spared in some cases but are often also sacrificed along with the deeper orbital tissues. A highly morbid procedure reserved for extensive and life-threatening orbital malignancies or infections.

Financial Disclosures None.

References

1. Cochran ML, Lopez MJ, Czyz CN. Anatomy, head and neck, eyelid. Treasure Island (FL): StatPearls Publishing; 2022.
2. Shumway CL, Motlagh M, Wade M. Anatomy, head and neck, orbit bones. Treasure Island (FL): StatPearls Publishing; 2022.
3. American Academy of Ophthalmology. Basic and clinical science course 2020–2021: oculofacial plastic and orbital surgery. San Francisco: American Academy of Ophthalmology; 2020.
4. Sajja K, Putterman AM. Müller's muscle conjunctival resection ptosis repair in the aesthetic patient. Saudi J Ophthalmol. 2011;25:51–60.
5. Rastrelli M, Tropea S, Rossi CR, Alaibac M. Melanoma: epidemiology, risk factors, pathogenesis, , diagnosis and classification. In Vivo. 2019;28:1005–11.
6. Reifler DM, Hornblass A. Squamous cell carcinoma of the eyelid. Surv Ophthalmol. 1986;30:349–65.
7. Kersten RC, Vagefi MR, Bartley GB. Orbital "blowout" fractures: time for a new paradigm. Ophthalmology. 2018;125:796–8.
8. Barrio-Barrio J, Sabater AL, Bonet-Farriol E, Velázquez-Villoria Á, Galofré JC. Graves' ophthalmopathy: VISA versus EUGOGO classification, assessment, and management. J Ophthalmol. 2015;2015:249125.
9. Bartley GB. The epidemiologic characteristics and clinical course of ophthalmopathy associated with autoimmune thyroid disease in Olmsted County, Minnesota. Trans Am Ophthalmol Soc. 1994;92:477–588.
10. Patel A, Yang H, Douglas RS. A new era in the treatment of thyroid eye disease. Am J Ophthalmol. 2019;208:281–8.
11. Hwang CJ, Eftekhari K. Teprotumumab: the first approved biologic for thyroid eye disease. Int Ophthalmol Clin. 2021;61:53–61.

Chapter 4
Anterior Segment: Cornea, Anterior Chamber, and Lens

Anh D. Bui, Tessnim R. Ahmad, Stephanie P. Chen, and Neel D. Pasricha

Cornea [1–10]

Introduction

- The cornea is the central, transparent portion of the anterior globe and is contiguous with the sclera at its periphery.

    - The sclera is the white outer shell of the globe and is covered by the conjunctiva, which extends from the cornea to the posterior face of the eyelids (Fig. 4.1).

- Transparency is ascribed to a highly ordered lamellar structure consisting of collagen fibrils, as well as due to a lack of blood vessels.

    - Corneal tissue obtains oxygen through diffusion from the tear film.

- Contributes two-thirds of the dioptric power (approximately 40D) of the human eye.
- Contains the highest density of nerve endings in the human body.

    - Intact sensation is crucial for the health and integrity of the cornea. Damage to corneal nerves can rapidly result in blindness.

A. D. Bui · T. R. Ahmad · S. P. Chen
Department of Ophthalmology, University of California, San Francisco,
San Francisco, CA, USA
e-mail: Anh.Bui@ucsf.edu; Tessnim.Ahmad@ucsf.edu; Stephanie.Chen2@ucsf.edu

N. D. Pasricha (✉)
Department of Ophthalmology, University of California, San Francisco,
San Francisco, CA, USA

UCSF Department of Ophthalmology, Wayne and Gladys Valley Center for Vision,
San Francisco, CA, USA
e-mail: Neel.Pasricha@ucsf.edu

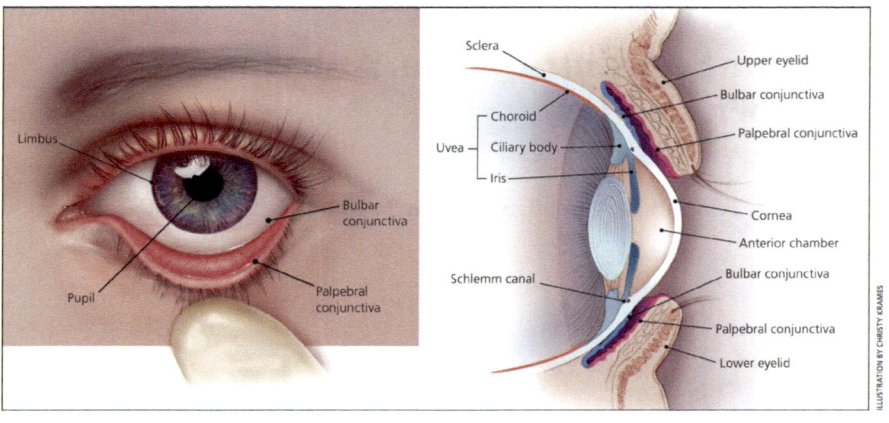

Fig. 4.1 The clear cornea is contiguous with the white sclera, which is covered by the transparent conjunctival membrane extending from the cornea to the undersides of the eyelids. [*Pflipsen M, Massaquoi M, Wolf S. Evaluation of the Painful Eye. Am Fam Physician. 2016 Jun 15;93(12):991–8. PMID: 27304768*]

Anatomy

- The cornea consists of five layers (Fig. 4.2).

  - Mnemonic to remember the layers: "ABCDE" (*A*nterior/Epithelium; *B*owman's layer; *C*orneal stroma; *D*escemet's membrane; *E*ndothelium).

Epithelium

- Tight junctions between epithelial cells form a key barrier preventing foreign material and pathogens from penetrating the cornea.
- Replenished by stem cells at the limbus (junction of cornea and sclera).

Bowman's Layer

- Acellular, non-regenerating layer composed of collagen fibers.
- Critical structural layer for the maintenance of corneal curvature.

Stroma

- Accounts for approximately 90% of the total corneal thickness.
- Composed of lamellae of type I collagen produced by keratocytes.

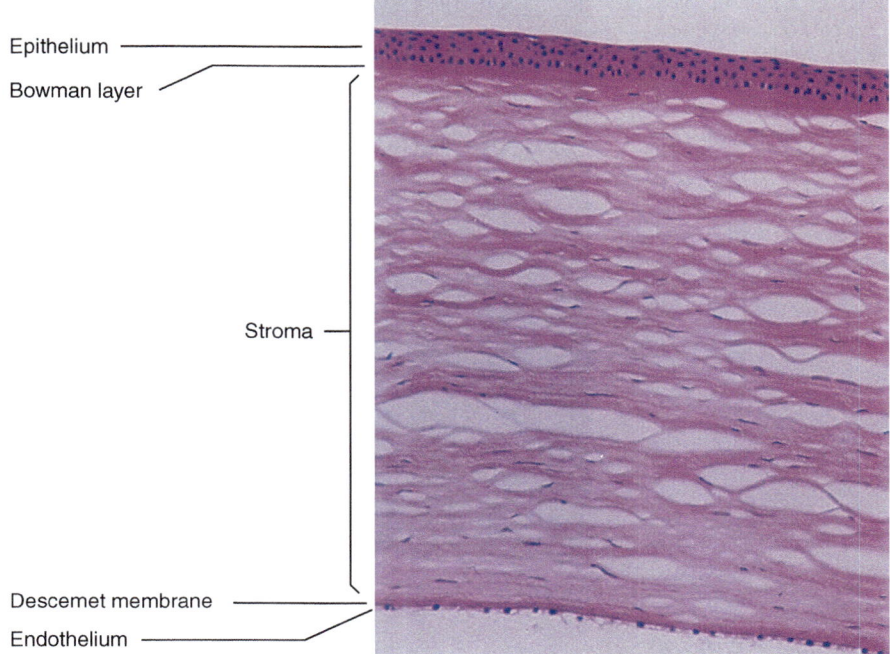

Epithelium

Bowman layer

Stroma

Descemet membrane

Endothelium

Fig. 4.2 The normal cornea is composed of five layers, including epithelium (4–6 cell layers thick), acellular Bowman layer, stroma, Descemet membrane, and non-regenerative endothelium. [*Source: BCSC 2021–2022, Figure 1-4, External Disease and Cornea*]

Descemet's Membrane

- Basement membrane of the endothelium.
- Synthesized by corneal endothelial cells and thickens with age (3 µm at birth, thickens to 10–12 µm in adulthood).

Endothelium

- Inner most layer of the cornea which is responsible for maintaining corneal transparency by dehydrating the corneal stroma. It acts to continuously pump ions and water back into the aqueous humor.
- The fixed number of cells at birth and the inability to regenerate lead to continuously decreasing endothelial cell density with age.

  – As endothelial cells are lost, the remaining cells enlarge and spread to cover deficient areas. When endothelial cell density is inadequate, the cornea becomes edematous less transparent resulting in loss of vision.

Fig. 4.3 A thin slit beam projected onto the cornea at a 45° angle is used to examine each corneal layer in cross-section. [*Source:* EyeRounds.org University of Iowa]

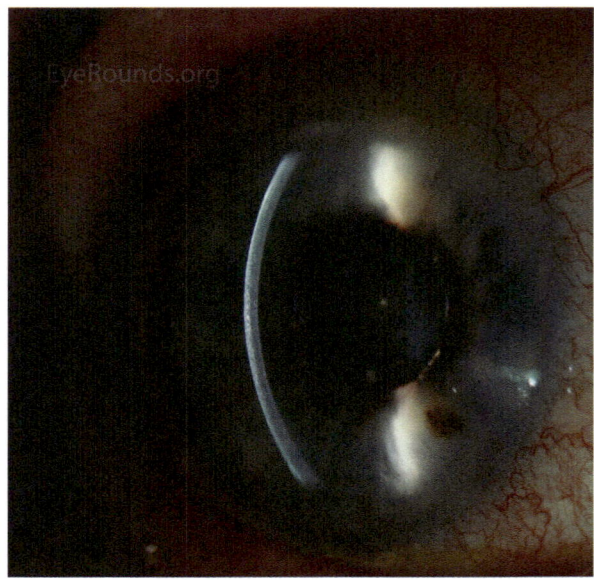

Fig. 4.3 A thin slit beam projected onto the cornea at a 45° angle is used to examine each corneal layer in cross-section. [*Source:* EyeRounds.org University of Iowa]

Physical Examination

- Use a thin slit beam at a 45° angle to examine the cornea in cross-section (Fig. 4.3).
- Assess corneal clarity and note the presence of any opacities.
- The use of fluorescein dye (stains disruptions of epithelial tight junctions) helps identify corneal abrasions/epithelial defects.

Pathology

Corneal Foreign Body

- Assess depth of corneal penetration (Fig. 4.4).
    - Deeply embedded foreign bodies may require removal in the controlled environment of the operating room under general anesthesia due to the risk of full-thickness injury and aqueous humor leakage.
- Rule out intraocular foreign bodies.
- Sweep the fornices and evert the upper eyelid to rule out for any conjunctival foreign bodies (Fig. 4.5).
    - Linear, vertical, fluorescein staining of the cornea may suggest a foreign body beneath the lid.

Fig. 4.4 A thin oblique slit beam demonstrates a metallic, hyperreflective, foreign body in the superficial cornea. [*Source:* EyeRounds.org University of Iowa]

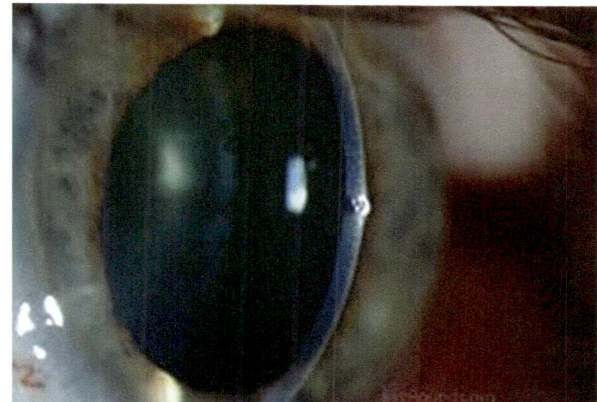

Fig. 4.5 Metallic foreign body that has become lodged in the palpebral conjunctiva lining the upper eyelid. [*Source: Stevens, S. How to evert the upper eyelid and remove a sub-tarsal foreign body. Community Eye Health. 2005 Oct; 18(55):110*]

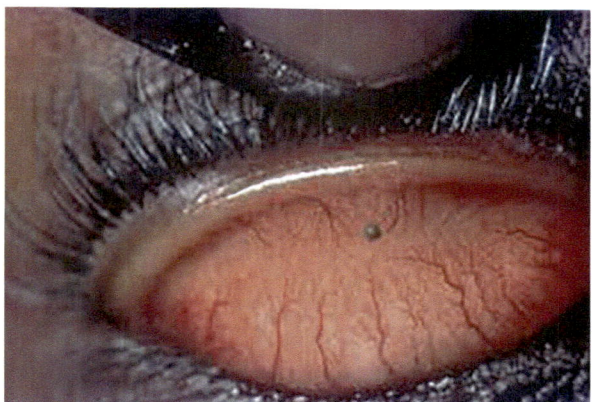

- Management:

  - Remove foreign body from cornea with a 30-gauge needle under direct visualization at the slit lamp.
  - Prophylactic topical antibiotic eyedrop while epithelial defect resolves.

Corneal Abrasion

- Corneal abrasions fluoresce bright green when illuminated with cobalt blue light after the application of fluorescein (Fig. 4.6).
- Opacification of underlying or surrounding corneal tissue suggests the presence of infection (**corneal ulcer**).
- Evert the upper eyelid to check for any conjunctival foreign bodies which may be causing the abrasion (Fig. 4.5).

Fig. 4.6 A corneal abrasion appears green under cobalt blue light after the application of topical fluorescein dye. [*Source: University of Iowa* EyeRounds.org]

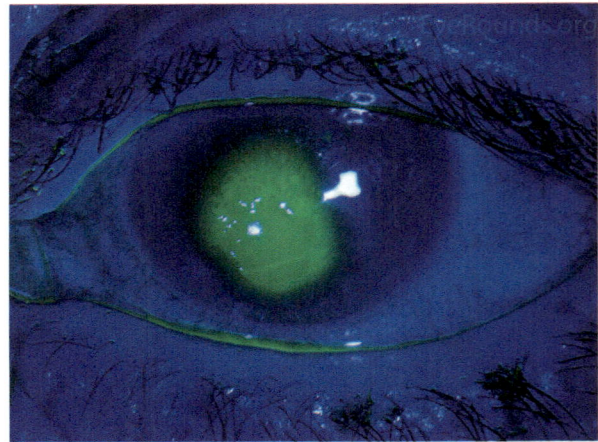

Fig. 4.7 Clinical appearance of a bacterial corneal ulcer with a dense white, nearly opaque, infiltrate surrounded by corneal edema. [*Source: BCSC 2021–2022, Figure 6-3, Ophthalmic Pathology and Intraocular Tumors*]

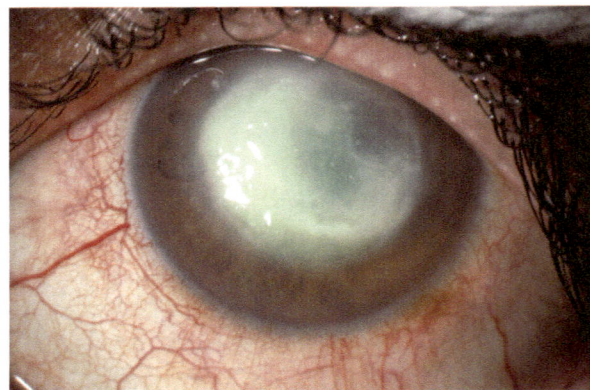

- Management:
    - Topical antibiotic eyedrop and/or ointment.
    - Consider topical cycloplegic agent for comfort.
    - Consider bandage contact lens for comfort (necessitates topical antibiotic while lens is in place).
    - Close follow-up for repeat examination while epithelium heals.

Corneal Ulcers

- Examination will typically show an epithelial defect associated with a whitish or opaque infiltrate surrounded by corneal edema (Fig. 4.7).
- Determine whether the patient has a history of contact lens wear.

    - *Pseudomonas aeruginosa* is the most common bacterial infection associated with contact lens wear, with an estimated annual incidence of 4–20 per 10,000 people.

- Risk factors include tap water exposure, trauma, or exposure to soil.

  - Tap water exposure is a risk factor for infection with *Acanthamoeba,* a free-living amoeba.
  - Post-traumatic eye infections are often caused by Gram-positive organisms, including *Staphylococcus, Bacillus, Streptococcus*, and *Enterococcus* species.
  - Penetrating eye trauma with a soil-contaminated foreign body can lead to an infection with *Bacillus cereus*, which can have devastating consequences.
  - Trauma involving vegetable matter, especially in tropical climates, can lead to fungal infections which require are often management challenges.

- Management:

  - Obtain cultures (bacterial, fungal, viral) by corneal scraping.
  - Broad-spectrum topical antibiotics (such as fortified vancomycin and tobramycin or moxifloxacin).
  - Avoid topical corticosteroids prior to obtaining a definitive culture diagnosis.

Corneal Laceration

- Corneal injury which penetrates the stroma or deeper structures.
- Examine with fluorescein to ensure the laceration is not full-thickness and leaking aqueous fluid (**Seidel test**) (Fig. 4.8).

  - A Seidel positive laceration is an ocular emergency and must be repaired immediately.

- Management:

  - Small (<2 mm) lacerations may be temporized with cyanoacrylate glue.
  - Large lacerations require operative repair with sutures in the operating room.

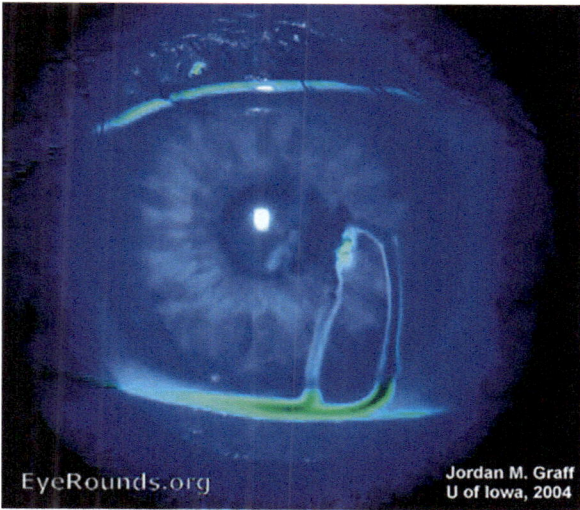

Fig. 4.8 Traumatic perforation of the cornea resulting in leakage of aqueous humor. In the Seidel test, a moistened fluorescein strip is applied to the area of the suspected leak. The fluorescein dilutes in the leaking aqueous humor, which fluoresces bright green and streams down the eye. This is a positive Seidel test. [*Source:* EyeRounds.org University of Iowa]

EyeRounds.org

Jordan M. Graff
U of Iowa, 2004

– Lowering intraocular pressure and reducing aqueous humor production with topical beta-blockers may reduce leaking and speed healing.

Herpes Simplex Virus Epithelial Keratitis

- Fluorescein staining shows characteristic corneal epithelial dendrites (Fig. 4.9).
- Management:
  – Oral antiviral medication (e.g., acyclovir, valacyclovir, famciclovir).

    Dose may need adjustment in patients with poor kidney function.

Chemical Injury

- Alkali burns are more serious than acid burns because they cause saponification of cell membranes, allowing the alkali agent to penetrate the eye.

  – Acids denature and precipitate proteins forming a barrier to penetration.
- Examine for corneal epithelial damage, corneal haze, and limbal ischemia (Fig. 4.10).
- Management:
  – Irrigate profusely with balanced saline solution (preferred) or water and check the ocular surface pH periodically. The eye should be irrigated until the pH is 7 (physiologic).
  – Never try to neutralize the chemical with another chemical substance as the exothermic reaction can lead to thermal injuries.
  – Sweep the upper and lower fornices thoroughly to remove any retained substance than can continue to damage the eye.

Fig. 4.9 Fluorescein brightly stains the base of the HSV corneal epithelial dendrites. [*Source: BCSC 2021–2022, Figure 11-8, External Disease and Cornea*]

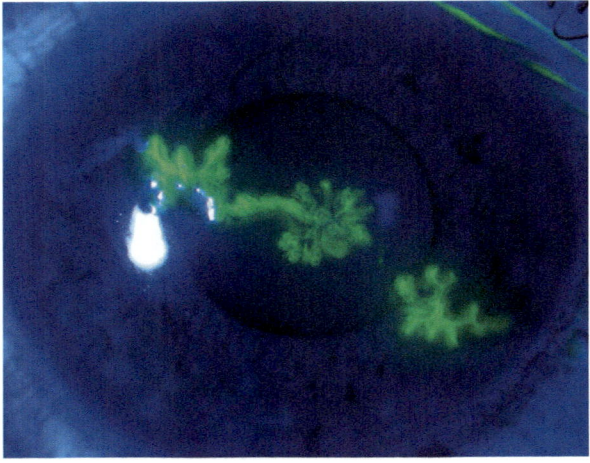

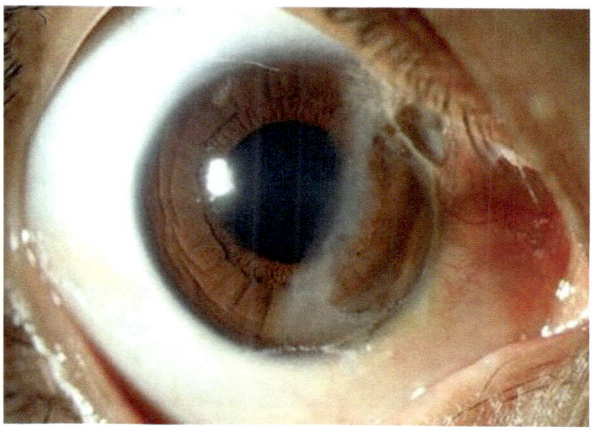

Fig. 4.10 Complete avascularity of the sclera following a chemical injury, note the abnormally white appearance and lack of fine conjunctival vessels. [*Source: Sharma N, Kaur M, Agarwal T, Sangwan VS, Vajpayee RB. Treatment of acute ocular chemical burns. Surv Ophthalmol. 2018 Mar-Apr;63(2):214–235. doi: 10.1016/j.survophthal.2017.09.005. Epub 2017 Sep 19. PMID: 28935121*]

- Administer topical antibiotic drops for prevention of superinfection, topical cycloplegic drops for comfort and topical corticosteroid drops to treat inflammation.

Dry Eye Syndrome [10]

- Dry eye is the most common eye condition and affects as much as 50% of the global population.
- Multifactorial disease characterized by impaired tear film homeostasis with resulting ocular symptoms.
- Associated with numerous systemic diseases, including mucous membrane pemphigoid, Sjogren's syndrome, and rosacea.

  - May have environmental triggers (e.g., pollution, allergens, low humidity) and can be eyelid-related (e.g., decreased blink rate from increased screen time, eyelid or eyelash malposition, incomplete eyelid closure).

- Eyelid may demonstrate meibomian gland disease, debris on eyelashes, or eyelid malposition. Fluorescein staining can show punctate epithelial erosions (Fig. 4.11), decreased tear breakup time, or decreased tear meniscus.
- Management:

  - Lubrication with artificial tears, gel, and/or ointment.
  - Warm compresses to heat meibomian glands and improve secretion.
  - Eyelid scrubs to clear debris and pathogens from the eyelashes.
  - Consider topical anti-inflammatory therapy in severe cases.

Fig. 4.11 Interpalpebral
punctate epithelial erosions
in a patient with dry eye
stained with fluorescein.
[*Source:* EyeRounds.org
University of Iowa]

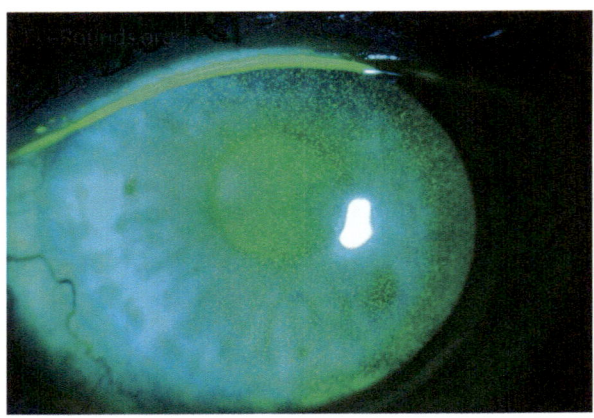

Anterior Chamber [3–6]

Anatomy

- Bounded anteriorly by the cornea and posteriorly by the iris (Fig. 4.12).
- Filled with **aqueous humor** which is primarily composed of water, albumin and other proteins, and glucose.
- The anterior chamber **angle** is located at the junction of the cornea and iris (Fig. 4.12).
  - The angle contains the major site of egress for aqueous fluid exiting the eye (**trabecular meshwork**) and is an important determinant of intraocular pressure.

Physical Examination

- Examine using a 1 × 1-mm slit beam on high intensity to look for any inflammatory cells or flare (caused by protein) present in the anterior chamber (Fig. 4.13).
- Examine for any red or white blood cells layering inferiorly in the anterior chamber.
- Determine depth of anterior chamber (shallow in angle closure glaucoma or globe rupture).

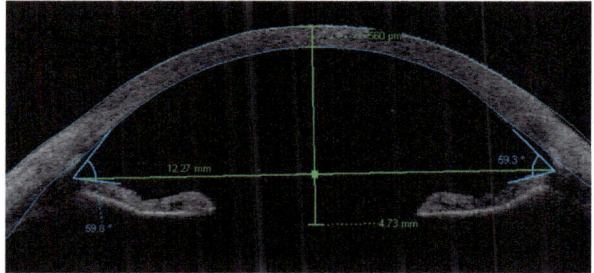

Fig. 4.12 Anterior segment optical coherence tomography (AS-OCT) demonstrating the anterior chamber in a phakic eye. The anterior chamber is bordered anteriorly by the cornea and posteriorly by the iris, with the angle located at their junction. In this case, the central anterior chamber depth is 2.73 mm. [*Source: BCSC 2021–2022, Figure 2-20, External Disease and Cornea (reproduced from Goins KM, Wagoner MD. Imaging the anterior segment. Focal Points: Clinical Modules for Ophthalmologists. American Academy of Ophthalmology; 2009, module 11)*]

Fig. 4.13 A small high intensity slit beam demonstrates inflammatory cells (left) and flare (protein, right) in the anterior chamber of a patient with anterior uveitis. [*Source: BCSC 2021–2022, Figures 5-1 and 5-2 (respectively), Uveitis and Ocular Inflammation*]

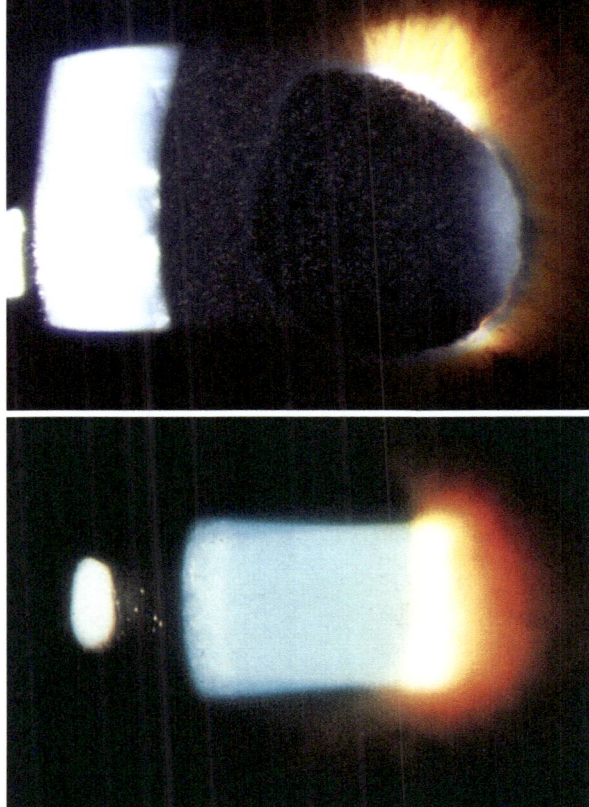

Pathology

Traumatic Iritis

- Inflammation of the iris, most commonly due to blunt trauma.
- Associated with photophobia, tearing, and decreased vision.
- Cell in the anterior chamber can be observed on slit lamp examination (Fig. 4.13).
- Management:

    - Cycloplegic agent for comfort and to prevent formation of **posterior synechiae** (adhesions between the iris and lens).
    - Topical corticosteroids to treat inflammation.

Traumatic Hyphema

- Accumulation of red blood cells in the anterior chamber (Fig. 4.14).

    - The bleeding originates from injury to vessels of the iris or ciliary body.

- May be associated with marked elevation in intraocular pressure if bleeding is sufficient to block flow through the trabecular meshwork.
- Highest risk of rebleeding is approximately 3–7 days after initial injury.
- Management:

    - Topical cycloplegia and corticosteroids.
    - Management of intraocular pressure.
    - Activity restrictions to prevent disturbance of organized clot.
    - Head elevation to facilitate inferior settling of blood cells.
    - Evaluate for sickle cell disease in at risk populations, sickled blood cells increase the risk of increased intraocular pressure and poor outcome.

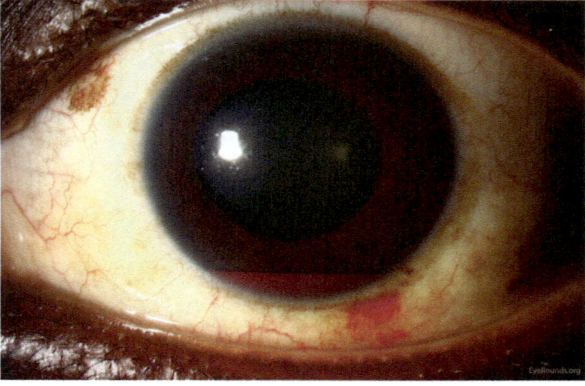

Fig. 4.14 Accumulation of red blood cells in the anterior chamber secondary to trauma. [*Source:* EyeRounds.org University of Iowa]

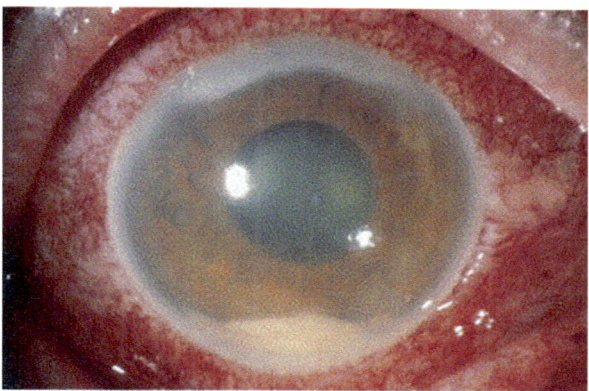

Fig. 4.15 Layer of white blood cells in the anterior chamber of a patient with uveitis. [*Source: Source: Anderson NG, Garcia-Valenzuela E, Martin DF. Hypopyon uveitis and relapsing polychondritis: a report of 2 patients and review of autoimmune hypopyon uveitis. Ophthalmology. 2004 Jun;111(6):1251–4. doi: 10.1016/j.ophtha.2003.09.026. PMID: 15177981*]

Hypopyon

- Layer of white blood cells in the anterior chamber (Fig. 4.15).
- Management:
    - Rule out endophthalmitis (infection) versus uveitis (sterile inflammation of the eye).
    - Sample aqueous humor for bacterial and fungal culture.
    - Topical antibiotics and cycloplegics.

Lens [3–6, 11]

Introduction

- Clear, biconvex structure between the iris and vitreous body (Fig. 4.16).
- Rapidly increases in thickness and curvature when transitioning from distance to near vision (and vice versa).

    - This process is called **accommodation** and the loss of this ability with age is termed **presbyopia**. This is why patients increasingly require reading glasses as they age.

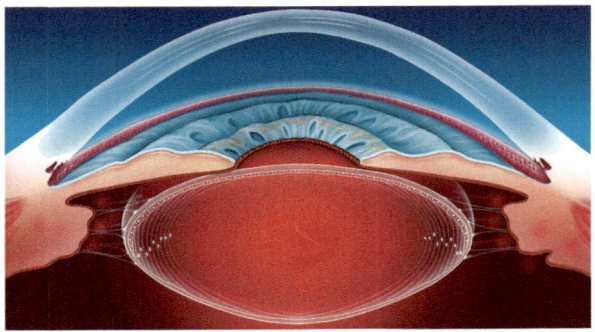

Fig. 4.16 Cross-section of the lens, a biconvex structure between the iris and vitreous body contributing approximately one-third of the refractive power of the human eye. [*Source: BCSC 2021–2022, Figure 2-1, Lens and Cataract*]

Anatomy

Capsule

- Outermost layer of the lens (Fig. 4.17).
- Basement membrane comprises type IV collagen.

Cortex

- Layer between the capsule and nucleus of the lens (Fig. 4.17).
- Comprises lens fiber cells after approximately age 20.
- Lower concentration of lens proteins, known as crystallins, compared to the nucleus.

Nucleus

- Central-most part of the lens (Fig. 4.17).
- Comprises lens fiber cells-long, thin, transparent cells that are continuously laid down by the lens epithelium for lifelong growth.

Physical Examination

- Examine for lens clarity and the presence of opacity (termed **cataract**).
- Examine for the type of lens in the eye.

  - Patients with natural lenses are **phakic**, while those with artificial lenses (i.e., following cataract surgery) are **pseudophakic** and those lacking a lens (after surgery or trauma) are **aphakic**.

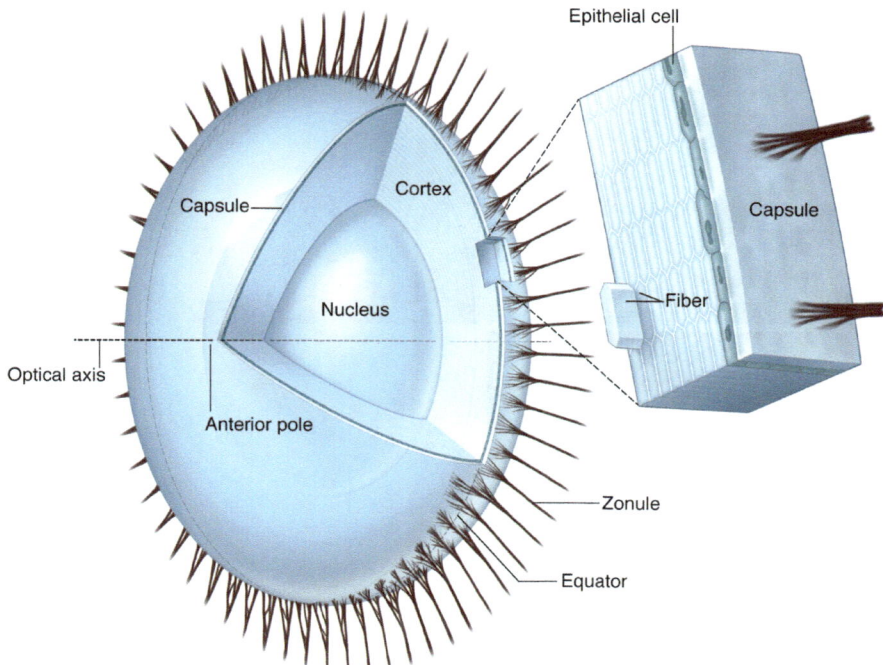

Fig. 4.17 The lens is composed of three main layers: the outer capsule, the central nucleus, and the intervening cortex. [*Source: BCSC 2021–2022, Figure 2-2, Lens and Cataract*]

Pathology

Cataract

- Three types of age-related cataracts: nuclear, cortical, and posterior subcapsular.
- Symptoms include myopic shift in refraction (increasing near sightedness), glare, halos, and decreased visual acuity.
- Can be seen on cross-section and retroillumination at the slit lamp microscope (Fig. 4.18).
- Management:
  - Initially can be managed with updated glasses or contact lens prescription.
  - Cataract extraction (e.g., phacoemulsification) with intraocular lens implantation is indicated once activities of daily living are impacted.

    Intraocular lens implants may be mono- or multifocal (theoretically allowing for clear distance and near vision without reading glasses) and may correct astigmatism (toric lenses).

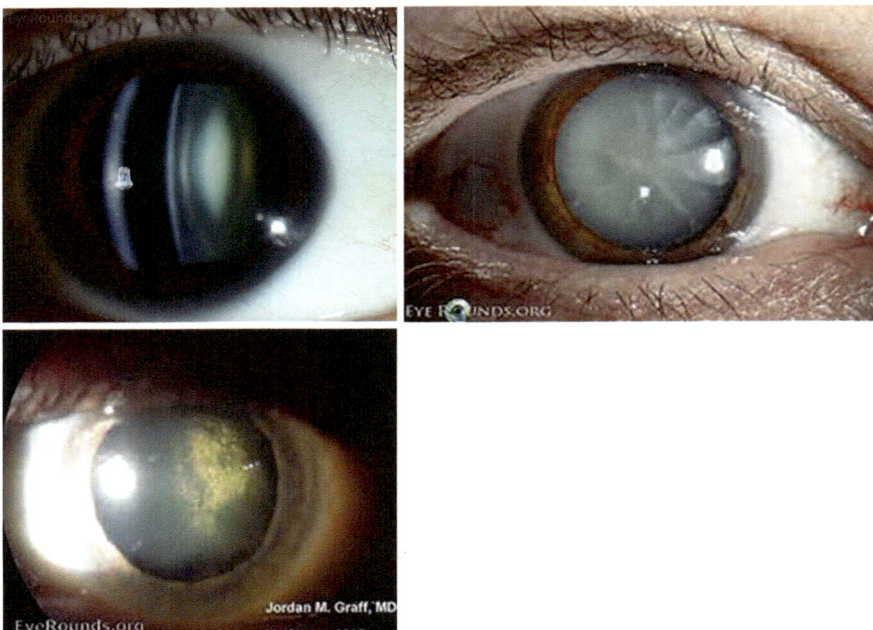

Fig. 4.18 Three major types of age-related cataracts include the nuclear sclerotic cataract (seen on cross-section), cortical cataract (seen with diffuse illumination), and posterior subcapsular cataract (seen with retroillumination). [*Source: University of Iowa* EyeRounds.org]

References

1. Mannis MJ, Holland EJ. Cornea. 5th ed. Amsterdam: Elsevier; 2021.
2. Krachmer JH, Palay DA. Cornea atlas. 3rd ed. Philadelphia: Saunders; 2013.
3. Root T. OphthoBook. Scotts Valley: CreateSpace Independent Publishing Platform; 2009.
4. Gervasio K, Peck T. The Wills eye manual: office and emergency room diagnosis and treatment of eye disease. 8th ed. New York: Lippincott; 2021.
5. Salmon JF. Kanski's clinical ophthalmology: a systematic approach. 9th ed. Amsterdam: Elsevier; 2019.
6. Allen RC, Harper RA. Basic ophthalmology: essentials for medical students. 10th ed. San Francisco: American Academy of Ophthalmology; 2016.
7. Rapuano CJ. Color atlas and synopsis of clinical ophthalmology: cornea. 3rd ed. New York: Lippincott; 2018.
8. American Academy of Ophthalmology. 2022–2023 Basic clinical and science course section 8: external disease and cornea. San Francisco: American Academy of Ophthalmology; 2022.
9. Poggio EC, Glynn RJ, Schein OD. The incidence of ulcerative keratitis among users of daily-wear and extended-wear soft contact lenses. N Engl J Med. 1989;321:779–83.
10. Craig JP, Nelson JD, Azar DT, et al. TFOS DEWS II report executive summary. Ocul Surf. 2017;15(4):802–12.
11. American Academy of Ophthalmology. 2022–2023 Basic clinical and science course section 11: lens and cataract. San Francisco: American Academy of Ophthalmology; 2022.

Chapter 5
Glaucoma

Elizabeth Bolton, Charles Miller, Russell Huang, and J. Minjy Kang

Introduction

- Glaucoma is the most common cause of irreversible blindness and the second most common cause of blindness worldwide [1, 2].
- The overall global prevalence of primary open angle glaucoma (OAG) in people over 40 years old is 2.4% and 9.2% in people over 80 years old [3].

Anatomy and Pathophysiology

- Glaucoma is a chronic progressive optic neuropathy characterized by apoptosis of retinal ganglion cells.
- The pathogenesis of glaucoma is multifactorial and involves damage to the axons of retinal ganglion cells at the level of the lamina cribrosa [4]. Loss of these neurons and their axons (which make up the retinal nerve fiber layer) causes the characteristic glaucomatous appearance of the optic nerve (optic nerve **cupping**) [1, 3] (Fig. 5.1).

E. Bolton · C. Miller · R. Huang · J. M. Kang (✉)
Department of Ophthalmology, Northwestern University Feinberg School of Medicine, Chicago, IL, USA
e-mail: elizabeth.bolton@northwestern.edu; elizabeth.bolton@nm.org; charles.miller@northwestern.edu; jessica.kang@nm.org

© The Author(s), under exclusive license to Springer Nature Switzerland AG 2023
E. Li, C. Bacorn (eds.), *Ophthalmology Clerkship*, Contemporary Surgical Clerkships, https://doi.org/10.1007/978-3-031-27327-8_5

Fig. 5.1 Glaucomatous optic nerve cupping. Fundus photo of optic nerve cupping, or an enlarged cup-to-disc ratio (the cup indicated by the dashed red arrow, the disc indicated by the black solid arrow)

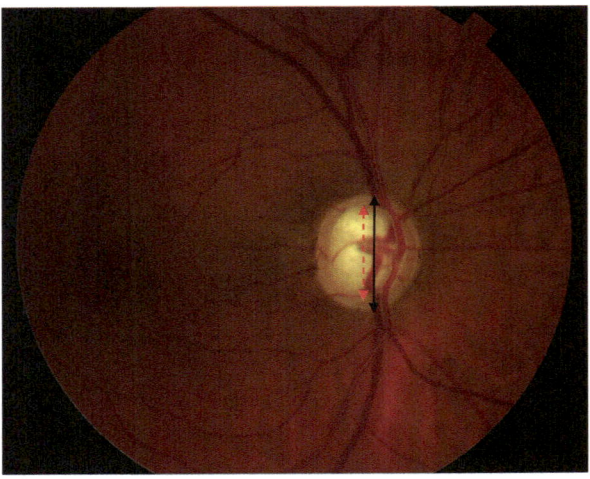

Aqueous Humor Production and Outflow

- The ciliary body is a smooth muscle located behind the iris and peripheral to the lens. It is composed of pigmented and nonpigmented epithelium [5, 6].
    - The nonpigmented epithelium is responsible for the production of aqueous humor, the fluid that fills the anterior chamber of the eye.
- **Intraocular pressure** (IOP) is determined by the rate of production of aqueous humor relative to its egress from the eye (Fig. 5.2).
- Inflow:
    - Aqueous humor is produced by active and passive secretion.
    - The secretion of aqueous humor is modulated through beta-2 receptors (stimulates secretion) and alpha-2 receptors (inhibits secretion).
    - Carbonic anhydrase is a key enzyme determining the rate of production of aqueous humor.
- Outflow:
    - Conventional pathway: 90% of aqueous humor leaves the eye through the pressure-dependent trabecular meshwork.

        Aqueous humor flows through trabecular meshwork to **Schlemm's canal**, through distal collector channels, and ultimately leaves the eye via episcleral vessels.
        Elevated episcleral venous pressure leads to reduced conventional outflow.

        This can be caused by venous obstruction (e.g., retrobulbar tumor, thrombosis of cavernous sinus or orbital vein) or arteriovenous anomalies (e.g., carotid-cavernous sinus fistulas, Sturge–Weber Syndrome).

        The highest point of resistance in this system is the juxtacanalicular tissue within the trabecular meshwork.

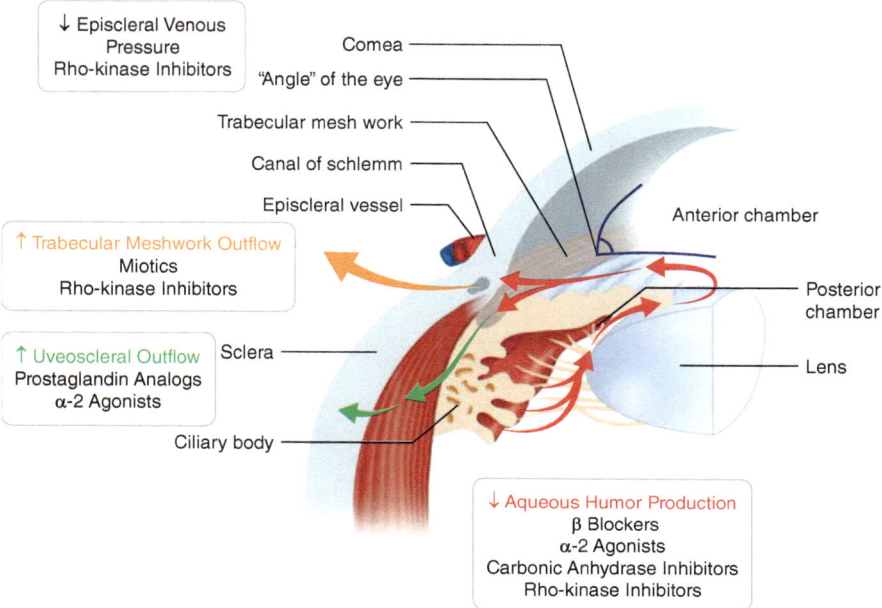

Fig. 5.2 Aqueous humor drainage pathways and mechanism of action of pharmacologic agents. Aqueous humor is produced by the ciliary body (red arrow). The majority of aqueous humor outflow occurs through the trabecular meshwork (orange arrow), with a small percentage of the outflow occurring through the uveoscleral tissue (green arrow). Intraocular pressure is determined by the balance of aqueous humor production, aqueous humor outflow, and episcleral venous pressure. The primary targets of different classes of glaucoma medications to lower intraocular pressure are depicted here

– Unconventional pathway: 10% of the aqueous humor leaves the eye via a pressure-independent mechanism.

  Fluid is passively filtered through intercellular spaces of the uveoscleral tissue [7, 8].

Optic Disc Anatomy

- The optic disc is formed by the coalescence of axons from the retinal ganglion cells (Fig. 5.3). The average vertical disc diameter is 1.88 mm and the average horizontal diameter is 1.77 mm.
- Axons traverse the porous structure of the **lamina cribrosa** as they course posteriorly to exit the globe.

  – It is at the level of the lamina cribrosa that glaucomatous damage occurs.

- The optic nerve is made up of greater than one million axons, one third of these fibers are responsible for the central 5° of the visual field [2, 7].

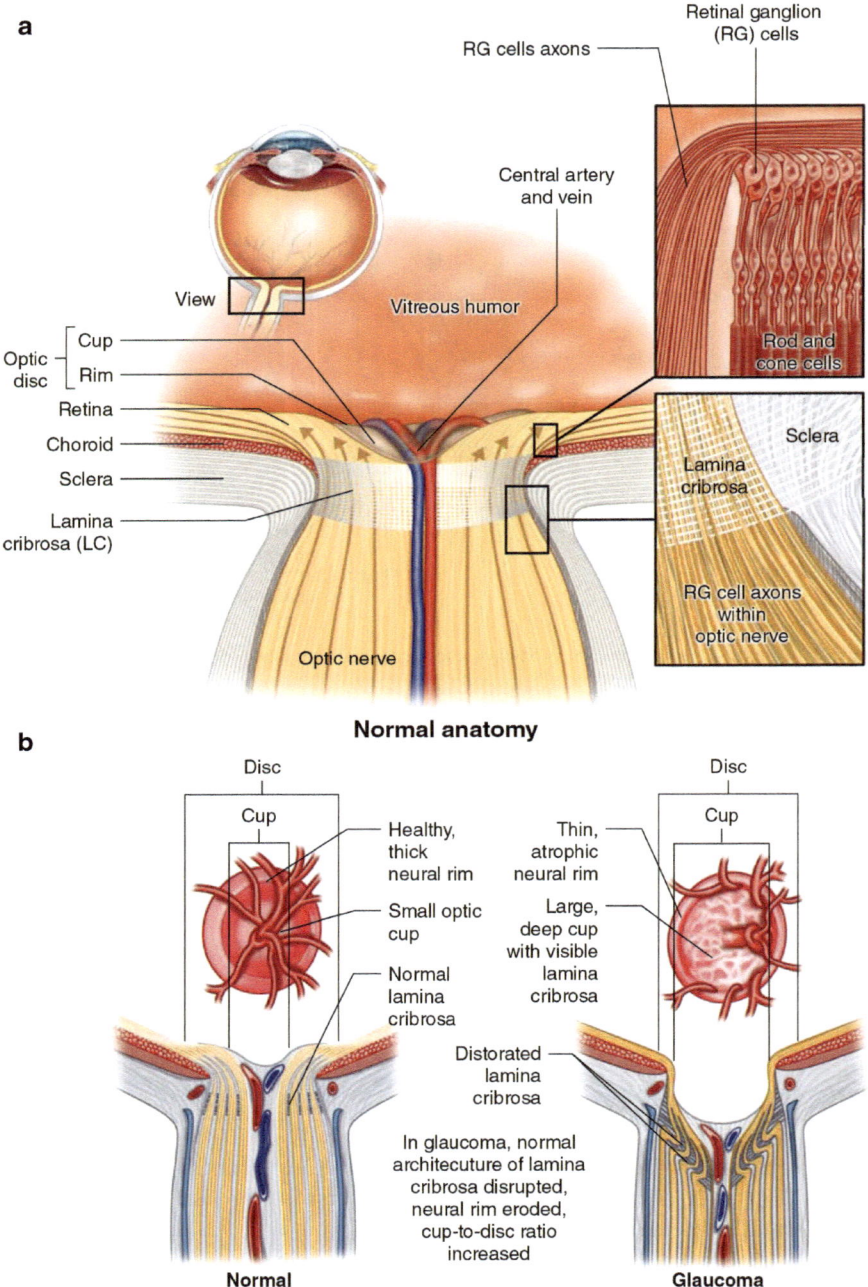

Fig. 5.3 Retinal nerve fiber layer and ganglion cell loss in glaucoma. In glaucoma, there is degeneration of retinal ganglion cells, which results in thinning of the neuroretinal rim tissue. On exam, this manifests as a larger cup to disc ratio of the optic nerve. The lamina cribrosa is also posteriorly displaced and thinned in glaucoma

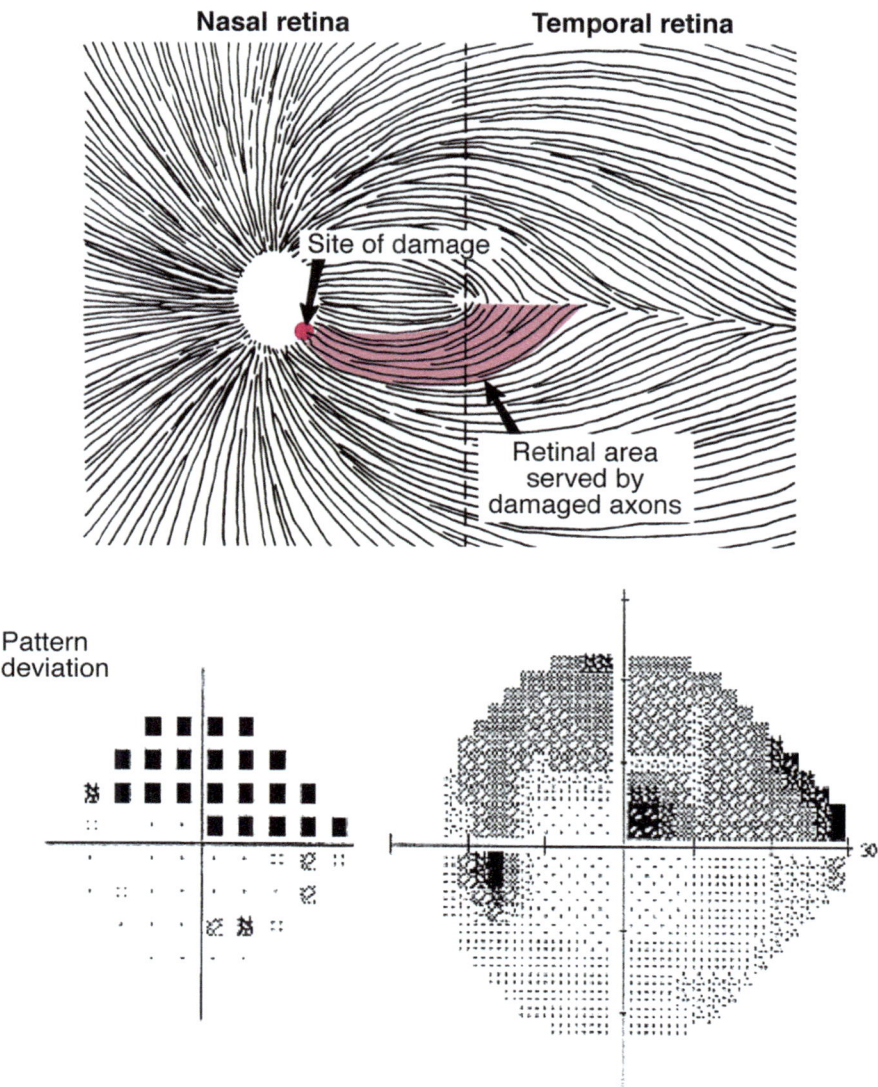

Fig. 5.4 Glaucomatous retinal nerve fiber damage and corresponding visual field defects. Glaucomatous damage to a nerve fiber bundle can lead to a corresponding arcuate defect in the visual field. Damage to the inferior optic nerve corresponds to a superior visual field defect. (Image Courtesy of AAO)

- Loss of neurons at the optic nerve head results in progressive visual field defects that classically respect the horizontal meridian (Fig. 5.4) [2, 7].

Intraocular Pressure

- The typical range of IOP in the general population is between 10 and 21 mmHg, with a mean of 16 mmHg. Elevated IOP (**ocular hypertension**) is a risk factor for glaucoma but is not pathognomonic for glaucoma. Low IOP (hypotony) refers to eye pressures of 5 mmHg and below.
- Different methods of contact and non-contact tonometry are used to measure the IOP. The gold standard of tonometry is **Goldmann applanation**.
- IOP can vary with positioning, the respiratory cycle (as a result of intrathoracic pressure), and the time of day (diurnal variation).

Classification

- Glaucoma is broadly categorized into "open" or "closed" angle glaucoma on the basis of the anatomic configuration of the **angle** (group of structures at the junction of the cornea, sclera, and iris).
  - The angle and trabecular meshwork are inspected with **gonioscopy**.

Open Angle Glaucoma

- Open angle glaucoma (OAG) is a chronic, progressive, optic neuropathy, typically with adult onset, and is the most common type of glaucoma.
- Risk factors for the development of OAG include increased IOP, older age, African race or Latino/Hispanic ethnicity, family history of glaucoma, thin central corneal thickness, and an increased cup-to-disc (C:D) ratio. Elevated IOP is the only modifiable risk factor.
- OAG is defined as either primary OAG, which has an idiopathic cause, or secondary OAG where an identified underlying condition drives the disease process.
  - Causes of secondary OAG are listed in Table 5.1 [9].

Closed Angle Glaucoma

- Closed angle glaucoma or angle closure glaucoma (ACG) is defined by physical obstruction of the trabecular meshwork, limiting conventional outflow, due to apposition or adhesion of the peripheral iris.
- Risk factors include female gender, older age, Inuit or East Asian ethnicity, a shallow anterior chamber, shorter axial length, and genetic factors [10].
- Acute ACG can lead to a sudden and significant IOP elevation and resultant corneal edema, nausea/vomiting, and pain.

Table 5.1 Types of secondary glaucoma

Name	Genetics/causes	Physical exam findings
Pseudoexfoliation glaucoma	LOXL1, deposition of fibrillar material throughout the eye including in trabecular meshwork	Exfoliative material on anterior lens capsule, on pupillary margin, iris transillumination defects
Pigment dispersion syndrome glaucoma	Zonular fibers of lens rub against the iris pigment epithelium. Pigment deposits on trabecular meshwork and lens capsule	Iris transillumination defects, pigment in anterior chamber, pigment on anterior lens capsule and corneal endothelium
Neovascular glaucoma	Ischemia or inflammation results in neovascularization of anterior chamber and angle and obstruction of the angle. Potential causes of neovascularization include diabetic retinopathy, central retinal vein/artery occlusion, chronic uveitis, intraocular tumors, ocular ischemic syndrome	Neovascularization of iris or the trabecular meshwork
Uveitic glaucoma	Chronic inflammation of the eye from uveitis can lead to secondary glaucoma from several mechanisms including edema/dysfunction of trabecular meshwork, inflammatory cells blocking trabecular meshwork, PAS blocking trabecular meshwork	Anterior chamber cell, keratic precipitates, posterior synechiae of the iris, PAS in the angle, neovascularization of iris/angle, iris bombe
Traumatic glaucoma	History of previous trauma to involved eye	Angle recession due to trauma or PAS in angle leading to angle closure
Steroid-induced glaucoma	Prolonged use of steroids (topical, intravenous, inhaled, or oral) can cause IOP elevation in susceptible patients	History of long-term use corticosteroids (particularly topical and periocular)
Drug-induced glaucoma	Medications that cause uveal effusion leading to secondary angle closure. Common culprits include topiramate, anti-depressants (e.g., bupropion), sulfonamides (e.g., acetazolamide, methazolamide), and sulfa antibiotics (e.g., Bactrim)	Sudden blurry vision due to acute myopic shift, eye pain, headache, narrow anterior chamber
Phacomorphic glaucoma	Mature lens causing anterior displacement of the iris and narrowing of the angle or obstruction of aqueous flow secondary to pupillary block	Mature cataract, narrow angle, fellow eye with normal anterior chamber depth

- Acute ACG is most often due to **pupillary block** (Fig. 5.5).
    - Pupillary block occurs when aqueous humor cannot pass through the space between the lens and the pupil margin. As a result, pressure increases in the posterior chamber and the peripheral iris balloons forward occluding the trabecular meshwork and limit conventional outflow.
- Pupillary block is more common in hyperopic (far-sighted) eyes due to the smaller and shallower anterior segment in these eyes [11].

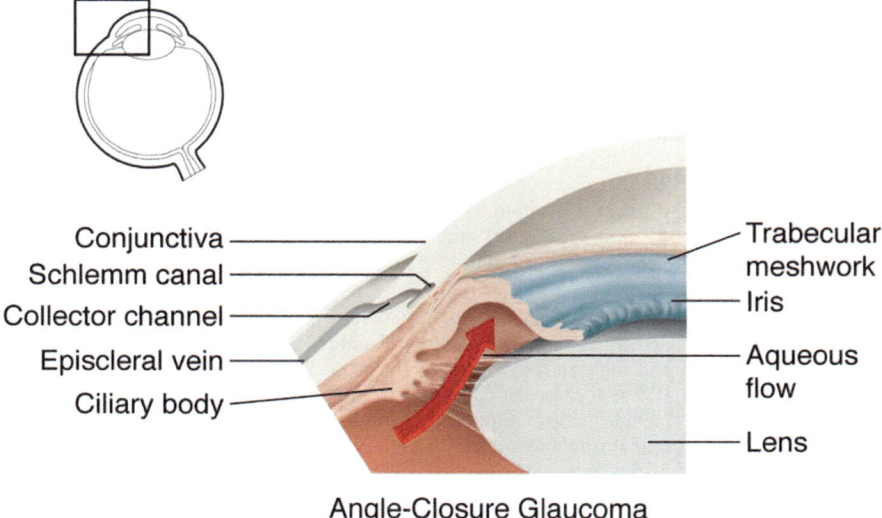

Angle-Closure Glaucoma

Fig. 5.5 Angle closure is often caused by pupillary block. In pupillary block, aqueous humor to flow from the ciliary body into the anterior chamber is blocked at the level of the iris-lens interface. Aqueous humor and pressure can then build up posterior to the iris, causing it to bow anteriorly into the iridocorneal angle and block the trabecular meshwork. (Image Courtesy of AAO)

- Other mechanisms of angle closure include:
  - Posterior pushing: The iris is displaced anteriorly by a posterior force resulting in angle closure. Examples include:

    Increased anterior–posterior lens diameter pushes the iris forward.
    A tumor or a benign mass, such as a ciliary body cyst, pushes the ciliary body and iris anteriorly.
    Plateau iris is an anatomic phenomenon in which the ciliary body is anteriorly rotated and as a result the iris projects forward narrowing the angle.

  - Anterior pulling: Anterior traction displaces the iris anteriorly leading to angle closure. Chronic iris contact can lead to the formation of **peripheral anterior synechiae** (PAS) which occlude the trabecular meshwork.

    Inflammation, neovascularization, and iridocorneal endothelial syndrome can all cause PAS.

Childhood Glaucoma

- Childhood glaucoma is an uncommon condition with an incidence of approximately 2.29 per 100,000 patients younger than 20 years old [12].

- Primary congenital glaucoma is diagnosed before age 4 and is associated with dysgenesis of the trabecular meshwork.
- Primary juvenile glaucoma is diagnosed after age 4 and before age 40 and is most often inherited as an autosomal dominant trait.
- Glaucoma following cataract surgery is a subtype of glaucoma that develops in young patients who have undergone cataract surgery early (congenital cataracts).
- Childhood secondary glaucomas are often associated with systemic conditions.

    - These conditions include congenital rubella, retinopathy of prematurity, Sturge–Weber syndrome, and Axenfeld–Rieger syndrome [12].

History and Physical

History

- Patient history should include:

    - Subjective description of vision (halos around lights).
    - History of any systemic medical problems.
    - History of trauma to the eye.
    - History of corticosteroid use.
    - List of systemic medications.
    - Associations: Raynaud's phenomenon, migraine history, sleep apnea, history of acute hypotensive episode, systemic hypertension or marked hypotension, diabetes, thyroid disorder.
    - Current and previous glaucoma medications.
    - Highest known IOP.
    - Previous history of medical therapy or laser or incisional glaucoma surgery.
    - Family history of glaucoma, macular degeneration, or retinal detachments.
    - History of activities associated with episodic episcleral venous pressure (EVP) elevation such as swimming with tight goggles, activities involving inversion, and playing wind instruments.

Physical Exam

- Visual acuity.
- Pupils: check for reactivity and for a relative afferent pupillary defect.

    - An eye in acute angle closure will have a mid-dilated, nonreactive pupil.
    - Glaucoma may result in an afferent pupillary defect if there is severe asymmetric glaucoma.

- IOP (Goldmann applanation preferred).
- Confrontation visual fields.

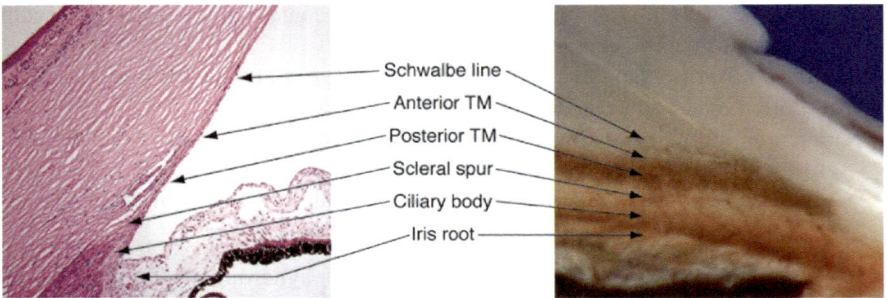

Schwalbe line
Anterior TM
Posterior TM
Scleral spur
Ciliary body
Iris root

Fig. 5.6 Gonioscopic image. Gonioscopic landmarks of a normal anterior chamber with histologic correlation. *TM* trabecular meshwork. (Image Courtesy of AAO)

- Color vision.
  - Asymmetry between the eyes could suggest an optic neuropathy other than glaucoma.
- Central corneal thickness (CCT) by pachymetry.
  - Average central corneal thickness is 540 ± 30 microns.
  - Thinner CCT is an independent risk factor for the development of glaucoma [13].
  - The thickness of the cornea can affect intraocular pressure readings measured by applanation.

    A thin CCT falsely depresses IOP readings.
    A thick CCT falsely elevates IOP readings.

- Gonioscopy is a procedure that assesses the angle between the iris and the cornea (Fig. 5.6) [14].
  - Observation of the angle through gonioscopy provides information on whether the angle is open (the trabecular meshwork in its entirety is visualized) or closed (the trabecular meshwork is not visualized).
  - If the trabecular meshwork is not seen, a goniolens is used to compress the cornea assess for the presence or absence of PAS.
    If the angle is not visualized after compression, closure due to PAS is presumed.
  - Abnormal blood vessels in the anterior chamber angle from neovascularization can be seen in neovascular glaucoma or chronic anterior uveitis.
  - The angle can also show a hyper deep configuration due to prior trauma (**angle recession**).

- Concavity or convexity of the iris on gonioscopy as well as hyperpigmentation of the structures visualized in the angle can represent certain secondary glaucomas including pigment dispersion syndrome or pseudoexfoliation syndrome.

Optic Nerve Evaluation

- Evaluation of the optic nerve head involves consideration of the size of the optic disc, the cup to disc (C:D) ratio, and the thickness of the neuroretinal rim.
- A stereoscopic assessment of the contour of the optic nerve at the slit lamp allows a subjective grading by the observer of the ratio of the cup (central depression without neural tissue) and disc (peripheral neural tissue). The size of the optic disc and any characteristics of the disc, such as sloping/notching or the presence of neovascularization or disc hemorrhages, are critical in the workup of glaucoma [2].
- Asymmetry of the C:D ratios greater than 0.2 or an individual C:D ratio greater than 0.7 are suspicious for glaucoma [2, 7].

Imaging

- Ancillary testing in glaucoma primarily involves monitoring for evidence of structural or functional disease progression.
- Structural progression is monitored with optic nerve imaging through optic disc photos and optical coherence tomography (OCT).

  - OCT imaging produces cross-sectional images of the optic nerve head and RNFL [15] (Fig. 5.7a, b).

    Detecting early RNFL thinning is important as it often precedes functional loss [16].

  - Optic disc photos are also useful in detecting progressive optic disc cupping.

- Functional progression of the disease is monitored with visual field testing.

- Standard automated perimetry (SAP) is a computerized visual field test which assesses visual function [17–19]. SAP involves displaying a light of a known size and intensity onto various areas of the visual field to systematically assess a patient's visual field. Typically the mid-peripheral (central 24 degrees) visual field is tested.

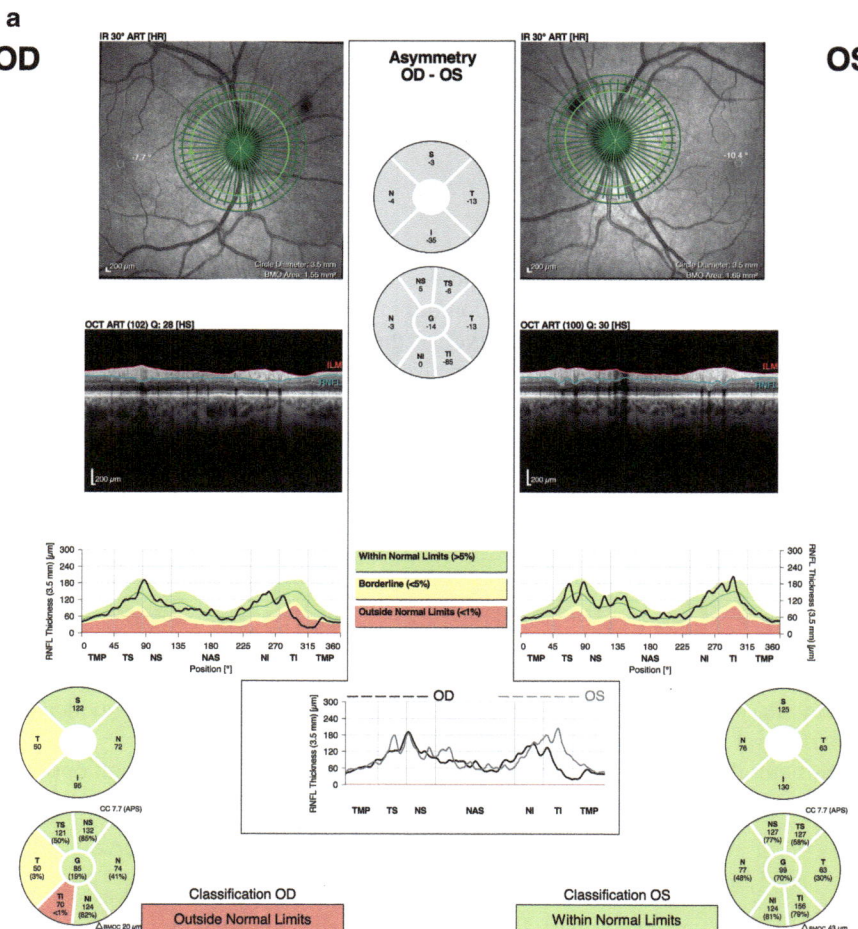

Fig. 5.7 A + B: OCT images of the optic nerve. (**a**) Demonstrates optical coherence tomography (OCT) showing retinal nerve fiber layer (RNFL) thickness of a right eye (OD) with inferotemporal RNFL damage due to glaucoma, and a left eye (OS) with healthy RNFL tissue. (**b**) Demonstrates progression of the inferotemporal RNFL thinning due to glaucoma over time

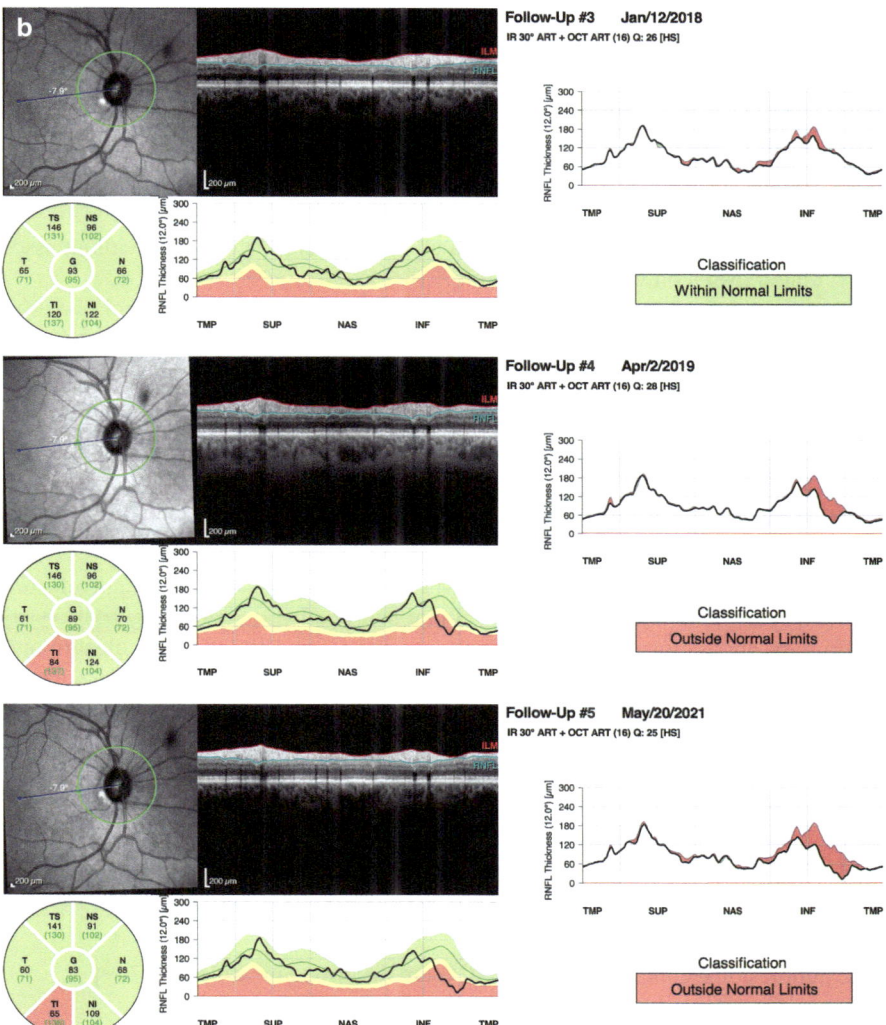

Fig. 5.7 (continued)

Diagnosis

Primary Open Angle Glaucoma

- The diagnosis of primary OAG is made in the setting of characteristic optic
  nerve head cupping with associated retinal ganglion cell layer loss and visual
  field changes. It is important to note that while an elevated IOP is often pres-

ent, it is not diagnostic. Many patients with glaucoma have untreated IOPs within the "normal" range of 10–21 mmHg (e.g., normal or low-tension glaucoma).

- Glaucoma suspects are patients who have one or more risk factors for glaucoma but do not meet the full diagnostic criteria. These include:

  - Ocular hypertension without glaucomatous optic nerve changes.
  - Family history of glaucoma.
  - An enlarged C:D ratio with associated retinal ganglion cell loss without associated losses on visual field testing.
  - A visual field defect that is not associated with any loss of retinal ganglion cell layer [2, 3, 9].

- Often patient require multiple assessments over time before a diagnosis of primary open angle glaucoma can be made.

Primary Angle Closure Glaucoma

- Primary angle closure suspects (PACS) are patients with >180° of angle closure without any PAS and no evidence of optic neuropathy.
- Primary angle closure (PAC) patients demonstrate >180° of angle closure and PAS or elevated IOP, but no optic neuropathy.
- Primary angle closure glaucoma (PACG) refers to patients with >180° of angle closure, elevated IOP, and evidence of optic neuropathy.
- Acute ACG is characterized by an occluded angle with symptomatically elevated IOP [9].

Secondary Open/Angle Closure Glaucoma

- Examples of secondary OAG and ACG are described in Table 5.1 [7, 9].

Treatment

General Treatment Principles

- IOP is the only modifiable risk factor and therefore the main target of treatment. For all types of glaucoma, lowering IOP has been shown to slow progression [2, 7, 9, 20].

  - Even in patients with low/normal tension glaucoma lowering IOP has been shown to be beneficial.

- There are different methods of IOP lowering including medications, laser treatment, and surgery.
- Treatment decisions should be individualized based on the patient's level of glaucomatous damage, general health, and preferences.

Medical Treatment

- Lowering IOP with medications can be done by decreasing aqueous humor production or increasing aqueous humor outflow (Table 5.2 and Fig. 5.2).

Table 5.2 Medications for treatment of glaucoma

Medication category	Examples	Mechanism of action	Side effects	Contraindications
Prostaglandin analogue	Latanoprost, Bimatoprost, Travoprost	Increase aqueous drainage through the uveoscleral pathway	Increased iris pigmentation, hyperpigmentation of periocular skin, lash growth, macular edema	Active uveitis (relative)
Beta blocker	Timolol	Decrease production of aqueous humor by the ciliary body	Bronchoconstriction, bradycardia	Pre-existing lung disease, including asthma/COPD, bradycardia (relative)
Alpha-2 agonist	Brimonidine Apraclonidine	Decrease production of aqueous humor by the ciliary body	Conjunctival hyperemia, eye irritation/allergy, central nervous system depression (infants and children)	Infants and children (absolute, **risk of central nervous system depression**)
Carbonic anhydrase inhibitor (topical)	Dorzolamide, Brinzolamide	Decrease production of aqueous humor by the ciliary body	Bitter after taste, eye irritation	Patients with sulfa allergy (relative) [21]
Rho kinase inhibitor	Netarsudil	Increased outflow through the trabecular meshwork, decreased aqueous production	Ocular irritation, injection	N/A
Carbonic anhydrase inhibitor (oral)	Acetazolamide Methazolamide	Decrease production of aqueous humor by the ciliary body	Paresthesias, GI upset, electrolyte imbalances, lethargy	Renal dysfunction (relative), impaired liver function, electrolyte imbalance

- Oral medication can be used when topical treatment is insufficient. They may be used for maintenance until surgery is performed or as long-term maintenance when surgery cannot be performed.

Laser Treatment

Laser Trabeculoplasty

- Mechanism: Selective laser trabeculoplasty (SLT) delivers laser energy to the trabecular meshwork. The exact mechanism is unknown, but it is hypothesized that the laser induces inflammation and remodeling of the trabecular meshwork leading to increased aqueous outflow [22].
- Indication: Treatment of OAG requires visualization of the trabecular meshwork. It is not effective in the treatment of ACG [23–25].

  – SLT is as effective as topical medical therapy and can be used as first-line therapy for the treatment of primary OAG [26]. SLT is especially effective for patients who have difficulty with instillation or adherence with topical therapy [23–25].

- Complications: IOP spike and inflammation after treatment.

Laser Peripheral Iridotomy (LPI)

- Mechanism: Laser creates a perforation in the peripheral iris allowing aqueous humor to bypass pupillary block and egress through the trabecular meshwork.
- Indication: LPI is first-line treatment for PACS, PAC, and PACG.

  – Patients with acute angle closure in one eye may benefit from prophylactic treatment of the fellow eye due to the risk of developing acute angle closure in the contralateral eye [27, 28].

- Complications: Inflammation, dysphotopsias/glare, and hyphema. Patients may also have persistently elevated IOP and require additional treatment [28].

Laser Cyclophotocoagulation (CPC)

- There are two types of CPC laser treatments: transscleral (TS-CPC) and endoscopic (ECP) [29, 30]. TS-CPC can be performed in the office or in an operating room and involves applying a probe to the external surface of the eye. ECP must be performed in the operating room and uses a probe that is inserted in the posterior chamber for direct visualization laser application to the ciliary body.
- Mechanism: Laser energy destroys the aqueous producing ciliary body epithelium.

- Indication: Refractory glaucoma, eyes with poor visual acuity or poor visual potential.
- Complications: Chronic anterior chamber inflammation, conjunctival burns (TS-CPC), hypotony, and vision loss.

Surgical Treatments

- There are three main categories of surgical treatment of glaucoma: minimally invasive glaucoma surgery (MIGS), tube shunt surgery, and trabeculectomy [2, 9, 31, 32].
- Lens extraction can be used to treat PAC and PACG in certain cases and can also be combined with other glaucoma surgeries listed above.

Minimally Invasive Glaucoma Surgery

- Mechanism: MIGS include a variety of surgical procedures and devices that work by increasing aqueous outflow through the trabecular meshwork by inserting a stent, excising trabecular meshwork tissue (goniotomy), or dilating the trabecular meshwork (viscodilation) [33, 34].
- Indication: Mild and moderate glaucoma.

  - Some MIGS devices are only approved in conjunction with cataract surgery.
  - Popular due to lower rates of complication and shorter surgical times compared to tube shunts and trabeculectomies [35]. However, they are not sufficient treatment in patients with advanced glaucoma who need very low IOPs.

- Complications: IOP spike after surgery, hyphema, need for revision [36].

Tube Shunt Surgeries

- Mechanism: Create a new drainage pathway for egress of aqueous humor, bypassing the trabecular meshwork. A tube is inserted beneath the conjunctiva into the anterior chamber to drain aqueous humor from the chamber into a plate that is secured to the posterior sclera. The two most commonly used tube shunt implants include the non-valved Baerveldt and valved Ahmed implant [3, 9, 31, 32].
- Indication: Treatment of moderate to severe glaucoma that is uncontrolled with medical therapy.
- Complications: Initial hypertensive phase after surgery (elevated IOP), a shallow anterior chamber, and conjunctival erosion by the plate [27, 32, 37].

Trabeculectomy

- Mechanism: Creates a new drainage pathway bypassing the trabecular meshwork. A hole is created in the sclera under a partial thickness scleral flap and aqueous is allowed to flow directly from the anterior chamber into a conjunctival **bleb** (an elevated segment of conjunctiva).
- Indication: Indicated for moderate to severe glaucoma that is uncontrolled with medical therapy.
- Complications: Cataract formation, vision loss, hypotony, and endophthalmitis.

  - Always at high risk of bleb infection and bleb leaks, which can lead to further complications and further surgeries [32, 38].

Lens Extraction

- Mechanism: Removal of the lens leads to a widening of the anterior chamber angle [37].
- Indication: PACG and PAC patients with IOP >30 mmHg.

  - May be more efficacious and cost-effective for the treatment of primary angle closure glaucoma than LPI [37].

- Complications: Intraocular hemorrhage, infection, retinal detachment, endophthalmitis [37].

References

1. Sihota R, Sidhu T, Dada T. The role of clinical examination of the optic nerve head in glaucoma today. Curr Opin Ophthalmol. 2021;32(2):83–91. https://doi.org/10.1097/ICU.0000000000000734.
2. Salmon J. Chapter 11: Glaucoma. In: Kanski's clinical ophthalmology. 9th ed. Amsterdam: Elsevier; 2021. https://www.us.elsevierhealth.com/kanskis-clinical-ophthalmology-9780702077111.html.
3. Zhang N, Wang J, Li Y, Jiang B. Prevalence of primary open angle glaucoma in the last 20 years: a meta-analysis and systematic review. Sci Rep. 2021;11:13762. https://doi.org/10.1038/s41598-021-92971-w.
4. Lamina cribrosa—American Academy of Ophthalmology. https://www.aao.org/image/lamina-cribrosa. Accessed 15 May 2022.
5. Anterior segment anatomy—American Academy of Ophthalmology. https://www.aao.org/image/anterior-segment-anatomy. Accessed 15 May 2022.
6. The 2 Layers of the ciliary epithelium. https://www.aao.org/bcscsnippetdetail.aspx?id=8f648b4f-3436-4ef3-bfea-672eb4aef10c. Accessed 15 May 2022.

7. Weinreb RN, Aung T, Medeiros FA. The pathophysiology and treatment of glaucoma: a review. JAMA. 2014;311(18):1901. https://doi.org/10.1001/JAMA.2014.3192.
8. Goel M, Picciani RG, Lee RK, Bhattacharya SK. Aqueous humor dynamics: a review. Open Ophthalmol J. 2010;4(1):52–9. https://doi.org/10.2174/1874364101004010052.
9. Tanna AP. American Academy of Ophthalmology 2021–2022 Basic and clinical science course, section 10: glaucoma. San Francisco: American Academy of Ophthalmology; 2020.
10. Amerasinghe N, Aung T. Angle-closure: risk factors, diagnosis and treatment. Prog Brain Res. 2008;173:31–45. https://doi.org/10.1016/S0079-6123(08)01104-7.
11. Angle-closure glaucoma—American Academy of Ophthalmology. https://www.aao.org/image/angleclosure-glaucoma-18. Accessed 15 May 2022.
12. Aponte EP, Diehl N, Mohney BG. Incidence and clinical characteristics of childhood glaucoma: a population-based study. Arch Ophthalmol. 2010;128(4):478–82. https://doi.org/10.1001/ARCHOPHTHALMOL.2010.41.
13. Extensive glaucomatous damage—American Academy of Ophthalmology. https://www.aao.org/image/extensive-glaucomatous-damage. Accessed 15 May 2022.
14. Gonioscopic landmarks—American Academy of Ophthalmology. https://www.aao.org/image/gonioscopic-landmarks. Accessed 15 May 2022.
15. Retinal nerve fiber layer—American Academy of Ophthalmology. https://www.aao.org/image/retinal-nerve-fiber-layer-2. Accessed 15 May 2022.
16. Sathyan P, Anitha S. Optical coherence tomography in glaucoma. J Curr Glaucoma Pract. 2012;6(1):1. https://doi.org/10.5005/JP-JOURNALS-10008-1099.
17. Heijl A, Patella VM, Bengstsson B. The field analyzer primer: excellent perimetry. 5th ed. Jena: Carl Zeiss Meditec, Incorporated; 2021.
18. Ballon BJ, Echelman DA, Shields MB, Ollie AR. Peripheral visual field testing in glaucoma by automated kinetic perimetry with the Humphrey field analyzer. Arch Ophthalmol. 1992;110(12):1730–2. https://doi.org/10.1001/ARCHOPHT.1992.01080240070033.
19. Bosworth CF, Sample PA, Johnson CA, Weinreb RN. Current practice with standard automated perimetry. Semin Ophthalmol. 2000;15(4):172–81. https://doi.org/10.3109/08820530009037869.
20. Anderson DR, Drance SM, Schulzer M, Collaborative Normal-Tension Glaucoma Study Group. Comparison of glaucomatous progression between untreated patients with normal-tension glaucoma and patients with therapeutically reduced intraocular pressures. Am J Ophthalmol. 1998;126(4):487–97. https://doi.org/10.1016/S0002-9394(98)00223-2.
21. Guedes GB, Karan A, Mayer HR, Shields MB. Evaluation of adverse events in self-reported sulfa-allergic patients using topical carbonic anhydrase inhibitors. J Ocul Pharmacol Ther. 2013;29(5):456–61. https://doi.org/10.1089/JOP.2012.0123.
22. Alvarado JA, Shifera AS. Progress towards understanding the functioning of the trabecular meshwork based on lessons from studies of laser trabeculoplasty. Br J Ophthalmol. 2010;94(11):1417–8. https://doi.org/10.1136/BJO.2010.182543.
23. Realini T. Selective laser trabeculoplasty. J Glaucoma. 2008;17(6):497–502. https://doi.org/10.1097/IJG.0B013E31817D2386.
24. Gazzard G, Konstantakopoulou E, Garway-Heath D, et al. Laser in glaucoma and ocular hypertension (LiGHT) trial. A multicentre, randomised controlled trial: design and methodology. Br J Ophthalmol. 2018;102(5):593–8. https://doi.org/10.1136/BJOPHTHALMOL-2017-310877.
25. Gazzard G, Konstantakopoulou E, Garway-Heath D, et al. Selective laser trabeculoplasty versus eye drops for first-line treatment of ocular hypertension and glaucoma (LiGHT): a multicentre randomised controlled trial. Lancet. 2019;393(10180):1505–16. https://doi.org/10.1016/S0140-6736(18)32213-X.
26. Gedde SJ, Vinod K, Wright MM, et al. Primary open-angle glaucoma preferred practice pattern®. Ophthalmology. 2021;128(1):P71–P150. https://doi.org/10.1016/J.OPHTHA.2020.10.022.

27. Radhakrishnan S, Chen PP, Junk AK, Nouri-Mahdavi K, Chen TC. Laser peripheral iridotomy in primary angle closure: a report by the American Academy of ophthalmology. Ophthalmology. 2018;125(7):1110–20. https://doi.org/10.1016/J.OPHTHA.2018.01.015.
28. Napier ML, Azuara-Blanco A. Changing patterns in treatment of angle closure glaucoma. Curr Opin Ophthalmol. 2018;29(2):130–4. https://doi.org/10.1097/ICU.0000000000000453.
29. Martin KRG, Broadway DC. Cyclodiode laser therapy for painful, blind glaucomatous eyes. Br J Ophthalmol. 2001;85(4):474–6. https://doi.org/10.1136/BJO.85.4.474.
30. Ansari E, Gandhewar J. Long-term efficacy and visual acuity following transscleral diode laser photocoagulation in cases of refractory and non-refractory glaucoma. Eye (Lond). 2007;21(7):936–40. https://doi.org/10.1038/SJ.EYE.6702345.
31. Lim R. The surgical management of glaucoma: a review. Clin Exp Ophthalmol. 2022;50(2):213–31. https://doi.org/10.1111/CEO.14028.
32. Gedde SJ, Feuer WJ, Lim KS, et al. Treatment outcomes in the primary tube versus trabeculectomy study after 3 years of follow-up. Ophthalmology. 2020;127(3):333–45. https://doi.org/10.1016/J.OPHTHA.2019.10.002.
33. Achiron A, Sharif N, Achiron RNO, Nisimov S, Burgansky-Eliash S. Micro-invasive glaucoma surgery: current perspectives and future directions. Curr Opin Ophthalmol. 2012;23(2):625–585. https://doi.org/10.1097/ICU.0B013E32834FF1E7.
34. Two approaches to MIGS: iStent and Trabectome—American Academy of Ophthalmology. https://www.aao.org/eyenet/article/two-approaches-to-migs-istent%2D%2Dtrabectome. Accessed 15 May 2022.
35. Mathew DJ, Buys YM. Minimally invasive glaucoma surgery: a critical appraisal of the literature. Annu Rev Vis Sci. 2020;6:47–89. https://doi.org/10.1146/ANNUREV-VISION-121219-081737.
36. Lavia C, Dallorto L, Maule M, Ceccarelli M, Fea AM. Minimally-invasive glaucoma surgeries (MIGS) for open angle glaucoma: a systematic review and meta-analysis. PLoS One. 2017;12(8):183142. https://doi.org/10.1371/JOURNAL.PONE.0183142.
37. Azuara-Blanco A, Burr J, Ramsay C, et al. Effectiveness of early lens extraction for the treatment of primary angle-closure glaucoma (EAGLE): a randomised controlled trial. Lancet (London, England). 2016;388(10052):1389–97. https://doi.org/10.1016/S0140-6736(16)30956-4.
38. Gedde SJ, Schiffman JC, Feuer WJ, Herndon LW, Brandt JD, Budenz DL. Treatment outcomes in the tube versus trabeculectomy (TVT) study after 5 years of follow-up. Am J Ophthalmol. 2012;153(5):803.e2. https://doi.org/10.1016/J.AJO.2011.10.026.

Chapter 6
Retina

Lauren Collwell, Sean Teebagy, and Karen Jeng-Miller

Introduction

The field of retina encompasses diseases of the vitreous and retina and their management. Conditions include some of the leading causes of blindness in the United States, such as diabetic retinopathy and age-related macular degeneration.

The path to sub-specialization in retina begins after undergoing ophthalmology residency. Training options include a medical (1 year) or surgical (2 year) retina fellowship.

- Medical retina focuses on non-surgical management of retinal diseases, including procedures such as intravitreal injections for macular degeneration or laser photocoagulation for retinal tears.
- Surgical retina encompasses medical retina but additionally utilizes surgical approaches to treat retinal pathology. For example, preforming pars plana vitrectomy for the treatment of retinal detachments.

Anatomy/Structures of the Posterior Segment

- **Optic nerve** (Fig. 6.1): Transmits electrical impulses from rods and cones to corresponding brain regions. The optic nerve contains only afferent (sensory) fibers. Optic nerve's diameter is 1.2–2.5 mm and contains 1.2–1.5 million nerve fiber layers [1].

L. Collwell · S. Teebagy · K. Jeng-Miller (✉)
Department of Ophthalmology and Visual Sciences, University of Massachusetts Chan Medical School, Worcester, MA, USA
e-mail: Colwell@umassmemorial.org; karenjeng@gmail.com

© The Author(s), under exclusive license to Springer Nature Switzerland AG 2023
E. Li, C. Bacorn (eds.), *Ophthalmology Clerkship*, Contemporary Surgical Clerkships, https://doi.org/10.1007/978-3-031-27327-8_6

Fig. 6.1 Fundus photography of the retina. A white dotted circle demarcates the area of the macula. The optic nerve is indicated with a white arrow. Arterioles (yellow arrow, smaller diameter vessel) and venules (yellow arrow, larger diameter vessel) provide blood flow in and out of the eye

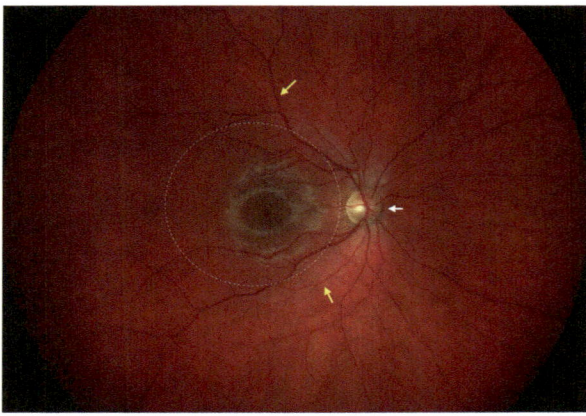

- **Arterioles/Venules** (Fig. 6.1): The central retinal artery, a branch of the ophthalmic artery, supplies the blood to the inner two-thirds of the retina [2]. The central ophthalmic vein drains blood from the retina to the cavernous sinus. The choroid supplies blood to the outer retina, including the photoreceptors, and drains into the vortex veins [3].
- **Retina**: The retina consists of ten concentric layers that convert light into chemical signals transmitted to the brain, which then interprets the signals to represent the three-dimensional world. Photoreceptors (rods and cones) are the key cells to convert light into a signal [4]. The **macula** (Fig. 6.1) is the part of the retina responsible for central vision and contains the **fovea**, which has the highest concentration of cones in the retina. The fovea is responsible for detecting fine details and color. In contrast, the peripheral retina is largely composed of rods, which function mostly in low light conditions. The anterior extent of the retina is the **ora serrata**, the junction between the choroid and ciliary body. Visualization of the ora serrata with indirect ophthalmoscopy often requires a technique called **scleral depression**.
- **Vitreous**: Gel-like substance inside the posterior segment composed of mostly type IV collagen. The vitreous fills the space between the lens and the retina. The vitreous base is the most anterior aspect of the vitreous gel and straddles the ora serrata. It is firmly adherent to the retina and ora at this location. The posterior hyaloid, the portion of the vitreous abutting the inner retina, is firmly adherent to the retina in the beginning stages of life, as the eye matures, liquefaction causes the posterior face to separate from the retina [5].
- **Choroid**: The choroid is a highly vascular layer of tissue that lies between the retina and sclera. It transports oxygen and nutrients to the outer retina.

Fig. 6.2 Optical coherence tomography demonstrating the layers of the retina

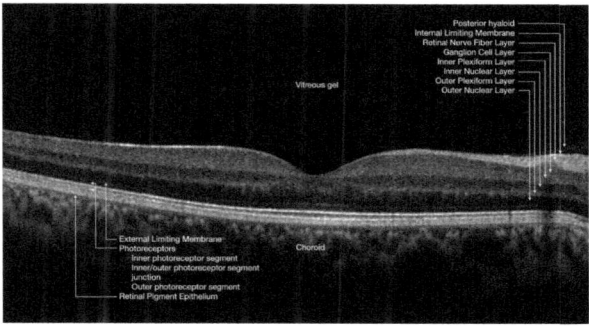

The Layers of the Retina [6]

Optical coherence tomography imaging offers a detailed view of the layers of the retina (Fig. 6.2).

- **Inner limiting membrane (ILM):** Basement membrane made up of footplates of Müller cells.
- **Nerve fiber layer (NFL):** Axons of ganglion cell bodies traveling to the optic nerve head. It is thickest proximal to the optic nerve and thinner distally.
- **Ganglion cell layer:** Cell bodies responsible for receiving inputs from the outer retina and transmitting this information to the brain via the axons of the optic nerve.
- **Inner plexiform layer:** Synapses between amacrine cells and retinal ganglion cells.
- **Inner nuclear layer:** Bipolar, amacrine, and horizontal cell bodies.
- **Outer plexiform layer:** Synapses between horizontal and photoreceptor cells.
- **Outer nuclear layer:** Photoreceptor cell bodies.
- **External limiting membrane:** Division between inner segments of photoreceptors from their cell nuclei.
- **Photoreceptors rods and cones:** Light sensitive tissue responsible for converting photons to chemical information transmissible to the inner retina.
- **Retinal pigment epithelium (RPE):** Pigmented cell layer outside of the neurosensory retina responsible for photoreceptor nourishment.

Exam Techniques

Retinal examination can be performed at the slit lamp and/or through use of a binocular indirect ophthalmoscope. Both approaches require condensing lenses to focus the image (Table 6.1).

Table 6.1 Different condensing lenses for ophthalmic examination

	Slip lamp lens			Indirect lens	
Lens	90	78	66	20	28
Suggested uses	Panretinal scanning	Macula and nerve	High detail	Panretinal scanning	Panretinal scanning, smaller pupil, larger field of view
Magnification	0.66 ×	0.77 ×	1 ×	~3 ×	~2.2 ×
Size of image compared to 2 mm slit beam	1.33 mm	1.1 mm	1 mm		

- Slit lamp

  - Slit lamp lenses are high plus power condensing lenses. They create an inverted view of the fundus. These lenses are often helpful when the eye has a small pupil.

- Indirect

  - Indirect lenses are used with indirect ophthalmoscopes. They also create an inverted view of the retina, but the field of view is larger and less magnified in comparison to the slit lamp lenses. The 28D lens is useful for small pupils and/or pediatric examinations because it provides a wider field of view than the 20D lens. The 20D lens provides a higher magnification in comparison to the 28D lens and is the standard lens used in adult indirect retinal exams.

- Scleral depression

  - Scleral depression is an important examination technique used to examine the far periphery of the retina. Due to the optics of the eye, the peripheral retina and ora serrata are often difficult to view with indirect ophthalmoscopy alone. During scleral depression, a smooth metal instrument applies gentle pressure on the sclera to indent the anterior aspects of the retina into the examiner's view. It also enables dynamic examination to provide three dimensional cues to elicit peripheral pathology, such as a retinal tear or hole.

Retinal Imaging [7]

- Optical coherence tomography (OCT): OCT is a noninvasive technology that uses light rays to provide cross-sectional views of the layers of the retina (Fig. 6.2). It provides a detailed view of microscopic pathology such as the pathologic markers of macular degeneration, drusen, (Fig. 6.3), or edema secondary to diabetic retinopathy (Fig. 6.4).
- OCT-angiography (OCT-A): OCT-A is a noninvasive imaging modality to examine the microvasculature of the retina and choroid (Fig. 6.5). It uses the movement of red blood cells to depict blood vessels, precluding the need for systemic

Fig. 6.3 Optical coherence tomography demonstrating drusen (red arrow), the pathologic markers of age-related macular degeneration. Also present is an epiretinal membrane (green arrow) which can distort the normal retinal contour

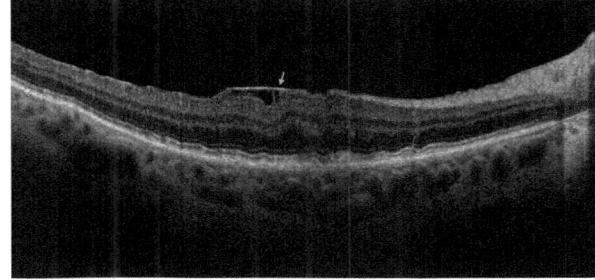

Fig. 6.4 Optical coherence tomography demonstrate intraretinal cystoid changes (blue star), termed diabetic macular edema, related to diabetic retinopathy

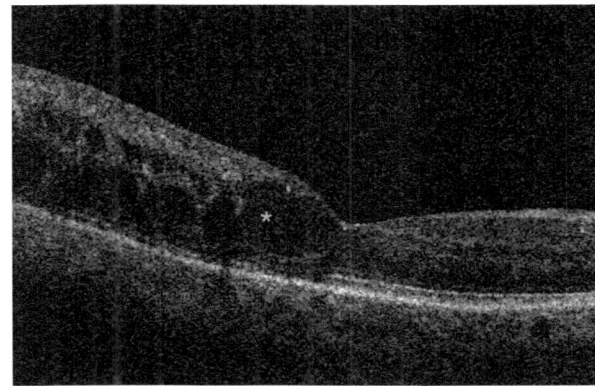

Fig. 6.5 Optical coherence tomography angiography demonstrating the vasculature through the superficial retina

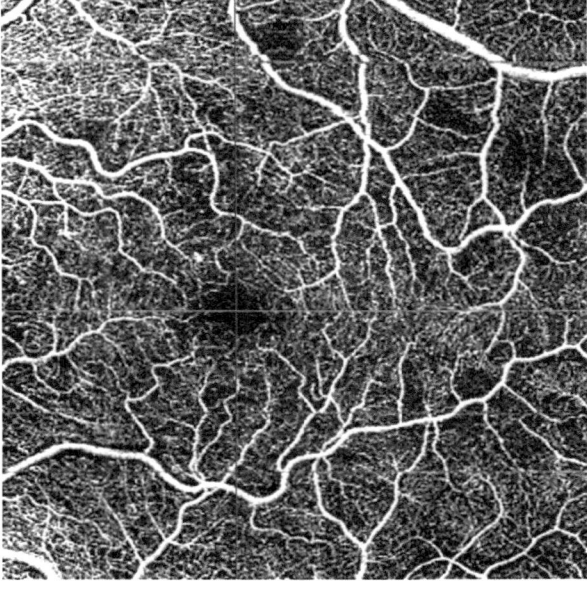

Fig. 6.6 B-scan of the eye demonstrating the vitreous cavity (pink star), retina (yellow star) and optic nerve (green star)

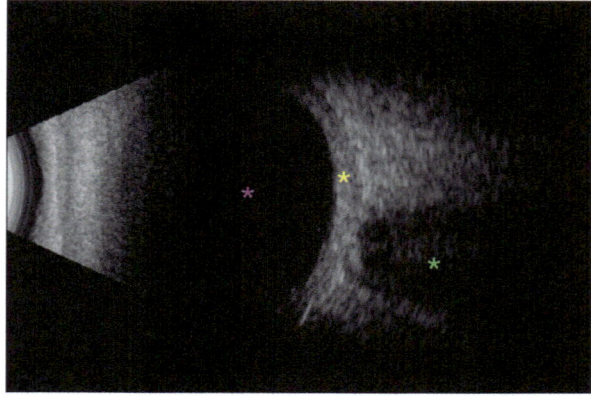

Fig. 6.7 Fluorescein angiography depicting peripheral nonperfusion (between the yellow lines) and microaneurysms (blue arrow)

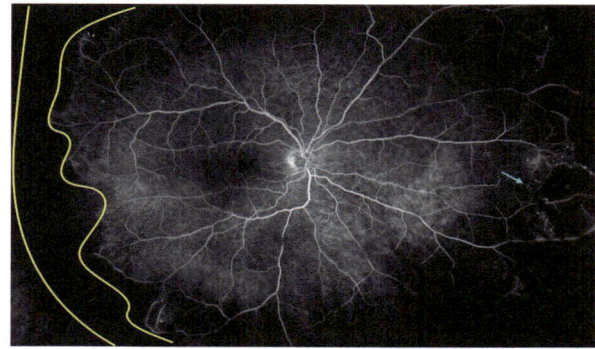

fluorescent dye administration. OCT-A is a noninvasive way to help detect choroidal neovascular membranes and evaluate areas of nonperfusion.

- B-scan: B-scan ultrasound measures the echogenicity of different tissues and represents this information as a two-dimensional brightness map. Hyperechoic tissues appear white (e.g., retina) while hypoechoic tissues appear less white or black (anechoic, e.g., vitreous) (Fig. 6.6). B-scans are useful in cases where media opacities (corneal opacification, dense cataracts) preclude adequate views of the retina with the indirect ophthalmoscope or slit lamp. They are also useful in characterizing posterior segment tumors, such as choroidal melanomas or metastases.
- Fluorescein angiography (FA): Fluorescein angiography is a photographic technique in which a fluorescent dye is introduced intravenously or orally to highlight retinal blood vessels (Fig. 6.7). It is particularly useful for the detection of retinal nonperfusion, vasculitis, and neovascularization.
- Indocyanine Green Angiography (ICG): Indocyanine Green Angiography, like fluorescein angiography, employs a systemic fluorescent dye to highlight vascular pathology. In contrast to FA, it is most useful in visualizing choroidal rather than retinal vasculature.
- Fundus Autofluorescence (FAF): Autofluorescence (Fig. 6.8) is a noninvasive imaging modality that does not require the use of invasive dyes. It utilizes the

Fig. 6.8 Fundus autofluorescence of the left eye. No abnormal autofluorescence patterns are detected

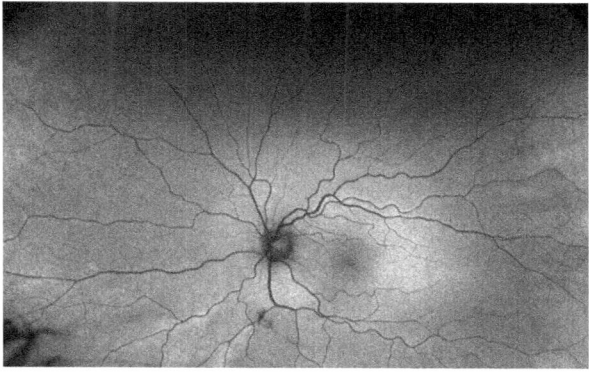

natural fluorescence properties of lipofuscin deposits in the retinal pigment epithelium to provide an image of the retina. This is important in diseases that lead to RPE dysfunction and lipofuscin accumulation.

High Yield Pathology and Treatment

- **Posterior Vitreous Detachment (PVD).**
    - Chief Complaint: New floaters and/or flashes.
    - Etiology: Vitreous liquefaction and syneresis resulting in vitreous condensation and separation from the retina.
    - History: Symptom onset and duration, quality and quantity of floaters, flashes of light, dark veil/curtain across visual field.
    - Differential Diagnosis: Ocular migraine, retinal tear and/or detachment, asteroid hyalosis, vitreous inflammation (infectious or noninfectious), vitreous hemorrhage.
    - Key Exam Findings: Central floater anterior to the optic nerve (**Weiss ring**) indicating separation of the vitreous from the optic disc.
    - Imaging Findings: OCT can definitively demonstrate and confirm the presence of a PVD (Fig. 6.9).
    - Treatment: An initial dilated exam with scleral depression. Repeat exam 4 weeks later to confirm no peripheral pathology is recommended. Retinal tears, holes, or detachments are treated when found.

- **Retinal Detachment (RD)**
    - Chief Complaint: Flashes, new floaters, shade/curtain across visual field.
    - Etiology: There are three types—rhegmatogenous, tractional, and exudative. Rhegmatogenous RDs, secondary to a retinal tear or hole, are the most common. Detachment of the neurosensory retina from its blood supply can quickly lead to permanent visual degradation.

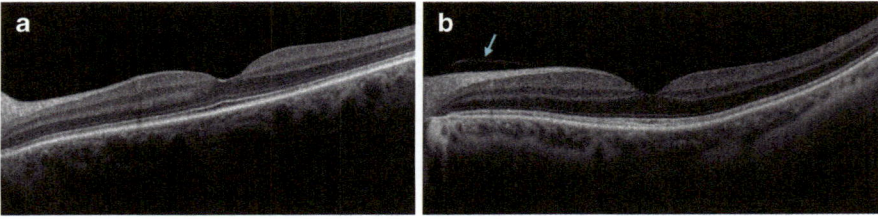

Fig. 6.9 OCT demonstrating (**a**) the presence of a posterior vitreous detachment and the (**b**) absence of a posterior vitreous detachment. The absence of a posterior vitreous detachment is primarily shown with persistent insertion of the posterior hyaloid onto the retina (blue arrow)

Fig. 6.10 A macula-involving retinal detachment from 7 o'clock with 11 o'clock with a tear at 9 o'clock (yellow arrow). OCT confirms the presence of subretinal fluid in the macula (inset photo, white star)

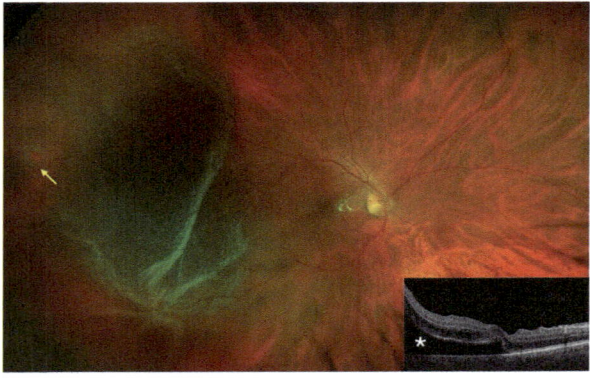

- History: Symptom onset and duration, trauma, family history of retinal tear/detachment.
- Differential Diagnosis: Retinoschisis, choroidal mass.
- Key Exam Findings: Pigmented cell in the anterior vitreous (**Schaeffer's sign**) and visible elevation and detachment of the retina from the underlying RPE. Important details to assess include (1) the lens status of the patient, (2) the presence or absence of a PVD, (3) the number of clock hours of retinal detachment extent, (4) all offending tears or holes and their locations, (5) the status of the macula.
- Imaging Findings: RD on fundus photography, subretinal fluid on OCT (Fig. 6.10).
- Treatment: Treatment can range from laser retinopexy (for small, peripheral asymptomatic retinal detachments), to pneumatic retinopexy, scleral buckle (encircling or segmental), or pars plana vitrectomy.

• **Diabetic Retinopathy**

- Chief Complaint: Decreased vision in a diabetic patient.
- Etiology: Microvascular damage to the structures of the eye due to long-term and/or uncontrolled diabetes.
- History: Year of diabetes mellitus diagnosis and type, last HbA1c, use of insulin, previous ophthalmic diagnoses and treatments.

- Differential Diagnosis: Ocular ischemic syndrome, branch or central retinal vein occlusion, hypertensive retinopathy, HIV-associated retinopathy, sickle cell retinopathy, radiation retinopathy.
- Key Exam Findings (Figs. 6.11 and 6.12, Table 6.2): Non-proliferative diabetic retinopathy findings include abnormally dilated small vessel outpouchings [called microaneurysms (MAs)], retinal dot blot hemorrhages (representing ruptured MAs), cotton wool spots (focal areas of ischemia), and yellow lipid and protein deposits (hard exudates). Macular edema can be present and is characterized by retinal thickening and hard exudates. Proliferative diabetic retinopathy includes all the findings of non-proliferative diabetic retinopathy but additionally demonstrates neovascularization of the iris, angle, optic nerve, or retinal periphery.
- Imaging Findings: OCT is very useful to detect macular edema. The main characteristics of macular edema in OCT include: increased retinal thickness, intraretinal spaces of hyporeflectivity, and flattening of the foveal depression (Fig. 6.4). Persistent macular edema can lead to Müller cell necrosis followed by formation of cystoid cavities within the retina.

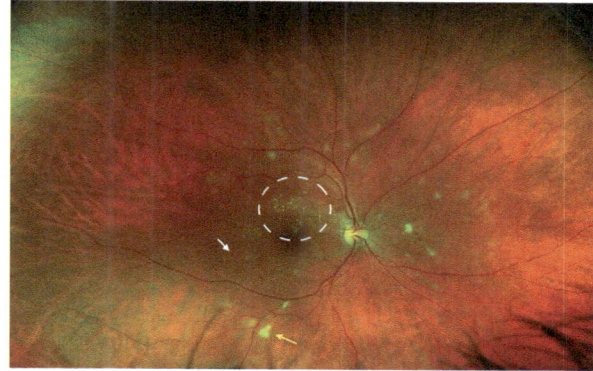

Fig. 6.11 Moderate non-proliferative diabetic retinopathy characterized by dot blot hemorrhages (white arrow), hard exudates (white circle), and cotton wool spots (yellow arrow)

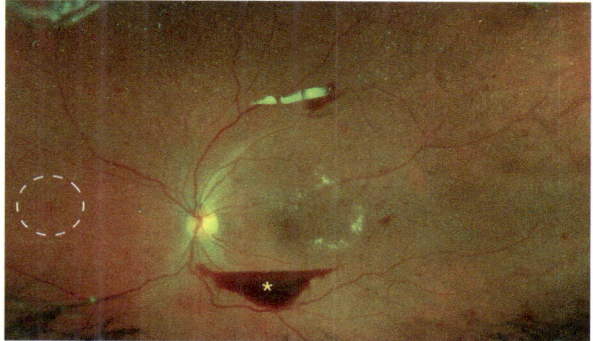

Fig. 6.12 Proliferative diabetic retinopathy with preretinal hemorrhage (yellow star) and retinal neovascularization (white circle)

Table 6.2 Stages of diabetic retinopathy [10]

Diabetic retinopathy category	Ocular findings
No retinopathy	No findings
Mild non-proliferative	Few microaneurysms (Mas)
Moderate non-proliferative	Many MAs, dot blot hemes (DBH), and/or venous beading, but does not meet severe stage. Cotton wool spots may also be present
Severe non-proliferative	4-2-1 rule: 4 quadrants of MAs and DBH 2 or more quadrants with venous beading 1 or more quadrants with intraretinal microvascular abnormalities (IRMAs)
Proliferative	Any neovascularization (NV) in the eye (iris, angle, optic disc, periphery)
High-risk proliferative	NV of the optic disc >¼ to one-third disc area Any NV of the optic disc associated with vitreous or preretinal hemorrhage Any NV of the retina associated with vitreous or preretinal hemorrhage

- Treatment: Treatment depends on the stage of disease. Once treatment is indicated, options to consider range from lasers (panretinal or focal), injections of anti-vascular endothelial growth factor (VEGF), injections of steroids, and/or surgery for non-clearing vitreous hemorrhages or diabetic tractional detachments [8, 9].

Age-Related Macular Degeneration (AMD)

- Chief Complaint: Asymptomatic, new blind spot, decreased vision, **metamorphopsia** (distorted vision).
- Etiology: AMD is categorized into dry (nonexudative) and wet (exudative) disease (Table 6.3). Dry AMD is characterized by drusen and atrophy. Wet AMD is defined by the presence of choroidal neovascular membranes. Decrease function of the choroid causes the accumulation of extracellular material (**drusen**) between the outer retina and choroid damaging the photoreceptors and leading to choroidal neovascularization (CNVM). Risk factors for AMD include advanced age, family history, smoking, and diet [11].
- History: Family history of AMD, smoking status.
- Differential Diagnosis: Drusen from normal aging, pattern dystrophy, drug toxicities.
- Key Exam Findings: Retinal drusen, retinal pigment epithelium changes/mottling, atrophy, hemorrhages, subretinal and/or intraretinal fluid.
- Imaging Findings: OCT is highly sensitive in detecting early pathologic findings of AMD (Fig. 6.3). These include drusen which can progress into atrophy and the

Table 6.3 Stages of AMD

AMD staging	Characteristics
Normal aging, no AMD	Few (<15), small (<63 µm) drusen without pigment changes, or no drusen
Early	Few intermediate-sized (63–124 µm) drusen with or without pigmentary changes
Intermediate	Many intermediate-sized drusen and/or one large (>125 µm) druse and/or geographic atrophy (GA) not involving the macula
Advanced non-exudative	GA involving the macula
Advanced exudative	Choroidal neovascularization

presence of CNVM which is usually represented by subretinal and/or intraretinal fluid.

- Treatment: Daily Amsler grid self-check at home to monitor for conversion of dry to wet disease, AREDS 2 vitamins to prevent progression to wet disease in certain patients, smoking cessation, and anti-VEGF injections for wet AMD.

Retina Procedures

Intravitreal Injection

- Localized medication administration minimizes undesired systemic effects and permits higher effective drug concentrations. Direct injection into the vitreous cavity bypasses the blood–ocular barrier and brings a drug in close physical proximity to intraocular structures, particularly the retina.
- Antibiotics, chemotherapeutics, and anti-VEGF agents are all routinely administered intravitreally. Viral vectors for gene therapy are another promising application for intravitreal therapy under active investigation.
- Risks of injection include endophthalmitis, traumatic cataract, retinal detachment, central retinal vein occlusion, and glaucoma. Proper technique and sterility minimize these risks.
- Injection is performed 3–4 mm posterior to the limbus, a landmark region overlying the pars plana. Entry within this safety zone minimizes the risk of puncturing the retina or lens.
- Vision is checked following injection to assess for potential complications. If vision is NLP, a central retinal artery occlusion secondary to ocular hypertension is likely and an anterior chamber paracentesis should be performed immediately to decrease intraocular pressure and restore retinal perfusion.

Pars Plana Vitrectomy

- Modern retinal surgery, like intravitreal injection, accesses the retina and posterior segment via the relative safety of the pars plana. Maneuvering instruments within the vitreous cavity can cause traction on the vitreous and tethered retina, risking iatrogenic retinal tears and detachment. As a result, vitreous removal (vitrectomy) to varying degrees is a general part of retinal surgery.
- Vitrectomy is accomplished by placing several trochars through the sclera at the pars plana. Instruments such as forceps, light pipes, or **vitrectors** are then placed into the posterior segment. The vitreous gel is then simultaneously cut and aspirated from the eye by the vitrector.
- Removal of the vitreous may be the end goal of surgery (as in cases of dense vitreous hemorrhage) or may facilitate additional surgeries such as repair of retinal detachments, removal of intraocular foreign bodies, or epiretinal membrane peel.
- Following successful vitrectomy, the vitreous cavity is often filled with saline, gas, or silicone oil to maintain a normal intraocular pressure.
- Indications for vitrectomy include rhegmatogenous or tractional retinal detachment, non-clearing vitreous hemorrhage, visually significant epiretinal membrane, macular hole, and endophthalmitis.
- Success rates with modern vitrectomy are high but complications may occur and include: endophthalmitis, retinal detachment, vitreous hemorrhage, and cataract.

References

1. Rapuano CJ, Stout JT, McCannel CA. 2020–2021 Basic and clinical science course (BCSC) section 10: glaucoma. San Francisco: American Academy of Ophthalmology; 2020. p. 59.
2. McCannel CA, Berrocal AM, Holder GE, Kim SJ, Leonard BC, Rosen RB, Spaide RF, Sun JK. 2020–2021 Basic and clinical science course (BCSC) section 12: retina. San Francisco: American Academy of Ophthalmology; 2020. p. 16.
3. Harris A, et al. Retinal and choroidal blood flow in health and disease. Retina. 2006;1:83–102. https://doi.org/10.1016/b978-0-323-02598-0.50011-2.
4. Neves G, Lagnado L. The retina. Curr Biol. 1999;9(18):R674–7.
5. Le Goff M, Bishop P. Adult vitreous structure and postnatal changes. Eye. 2008;22:1214–22.
6. Kolb H. Simple anatomy of the retina. In: Kolb H, et al., editors. Webvision: The organization of the retina and visual system. University of Utah Health Sciences Center; 2005.
7. Keane PA, Sadda SR. Retinal imaging in the twenty-first century: state of the art and future directions. Ophthalmology. 2014;121(12):2489–500.
8. Aiello LM. Perspectives on diabetic retinopathy. Am J Ophthalmol. 2003;136:122.
9. Stitt AW, Curtis TM, Chen M, Medina RJ, et al. The progress in understanding and treatment of diabetic retinopathy. Prog Retin Eye Res. 2016;51:156–86.
10. Early Treatment Diabetic Retinopathy Study Research Group. Grading diabetic retinopathy from stereoscopic color fundus photographs—an extension of the modified Airlie House classification. ETDRS report number 10. Ophthalmology. 1991;98(5 Suppl):786–806.
11. Age-Related Eye Disease Study Research Group. The Age-Related Eye Disease Study (AREDS): design implications. AREDS report no. 1. Control Clin Trials. 1999;20(6):573–600. https://doi.org/10.1016/s0197-2456(99)00031-8.

Chapter 7
Uveitis

Jacob S. Heng and Ninani Kombo

Anatomy

The uveal tract is classically divided into three parts arranged from anterior to posterior:

- Iris
- Ciliary body
- Choroid

Uveitis may be classified according to the anatomic site of inflammation and time course (Fig. 7.1). It may also be useful to classify uveitis on the basis of etiology as indicated in Table 7.1.

J. S. Heng · N. Kombo (✉)
Department of Ophthalmology and Visual Science, Yale School of Medicine, New Haven, CT, USA
e-mail: jacob.heng@yale.edu; ninani.kombo@yale.edu

Fig. 7.1 Classification of uveitis into anterior, intermediate, and posterior uveitis (bold) according to anatomic site affected. Relevant structures of the eye are indicated. The corresponding parts of the uveal tract are indicated in italics

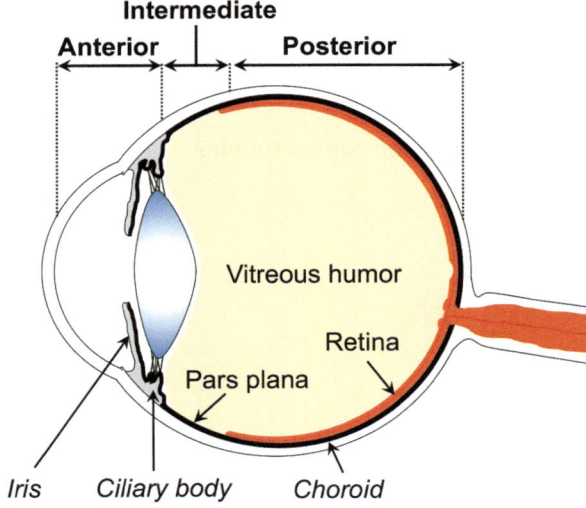

Table 7.1 IUSG clinical classification of uveitis

Etiology	Includes
Infectious	Bacterial Viral Fungal Parasitic Others
Non-infectious	Known systemic associations No known systemic associations
Masquerade	Neoplastic Non-neoplastic

Epidemiology

Uveitis is a relatively uncommon disease with an incidence of approximately 50 per 100,000 people per year and a prevalence of 150 per 100,000 [1]. Although uveitis is relatively rare it one of the leading causes of blindness in the developed world [2]. Up to 70% of patients with uveitis will experience some degree of vision loss and more than 10% of affected patients will experience significant vision loss and blindness [3]. The incidence of uveitis increases with age [1] and is more common in women than in men [4]. Anterior uveitis is the most common subtype and accounts for 80% of cases in the United States [5].

History

Key components of history include the onset and duration of symptoms. Uveitis may be subcategorized based on this information.

- Acute—sudden onset and limited duration.
- Recurrent—repeated episodes separated by periods of inactivity without treatment >3 months in duration.
- Chronic—persistent uveitis with relapse <3 months after discontinuing treatment.

Common symptoms vary depending on the site of inflammation and include:

- Anterior uveitis—pain, injection, photophobia, decreased vision.
- Intermediate uveitis—floaters, decreased vision.
- Posterior uveitis—floaters, photopsias, scotomas, decreased vision, **metamorphopsia** (distortion of straight lines).

Pain and injection typically result from inflammation of the iris and anterior chamber. Pain and photophobia are predominantly due to ciliary spasm and inflammation of the muscles of the iris. However, pain may also result from increased intraocular pressure.

- Juvenile idiopathic arthritis is a notable exception classically characterized by painless anterior uveitis.

Decreased visual acuity may be caused by inflammatory cells or debris in the visual axis or as a result of the sequela of chronic inflammation such as cataract or band keratopathy. Macular edema may also cause decreased visual acuity and may be present in posterior and intermediate uveitis.

Exam

A comprehensive physical examination is essential in determining the underlying etiology of uveitis. This exam is not limited to the eye as uveitis is frequently a manifestation of systemic disease.

- Skin—Rash, vitiligo, nodules
- Conjunctiva/Sclera—Injection, scleral thinning
- Cornea—Band keratopathy, keratic precipitates, endothelial pigment
- Anterior Chamber—Cell, flare, fibrin, hypopyon (Fig. 7.2)
- Iris—Posterior synechiae (Fig. 7.3), transillumination defects, heterochromia
- Lens—Cataract
- Vitreous—Inflammatory cells (Fig. 7.4), snowballs, or snowbanks (Fig. 7.5)
- Retina—Cellular infiltrates (Fig. 7.3), perivascular cuffing (Fig. 7.6a, b), edema, neovascularization
- Optic nerve—Edema, neovascularization

Fig. 7.2 Injection
associated with acute
anterior uveitis

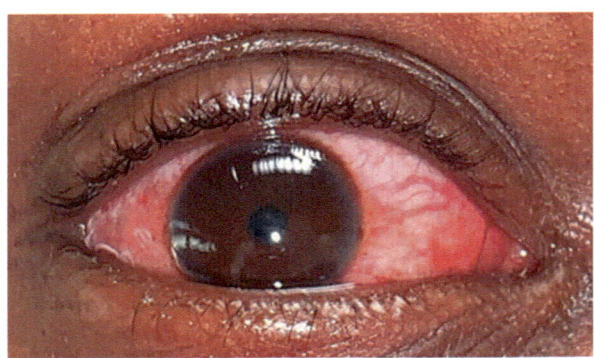

Fig. 7.3 HLA-B27
associated anterior uveitis
demonstrating hypopyon
and posterior synechiae

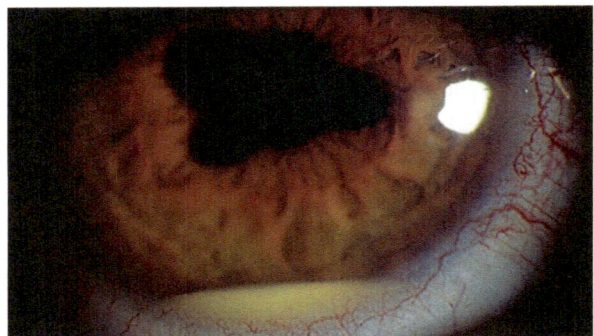

Fig. 7.4 Toxoplasmosis
chorioretinitis
demonstrating vitritis
(hazy view of posterior
segment structures) and
underlying chorioretinal
inflammation (white lesion
superiorly)

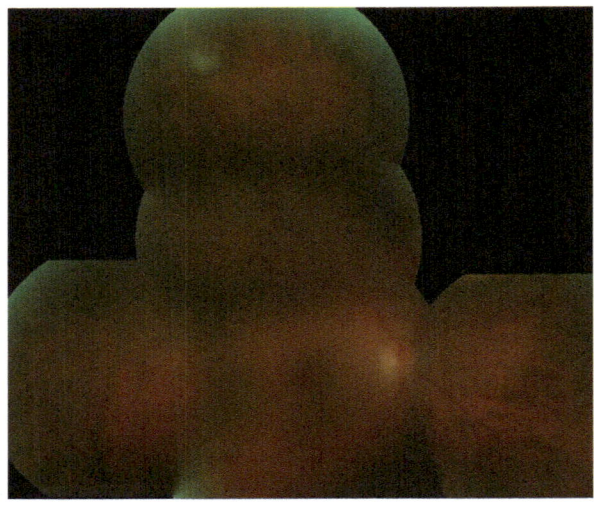

The slit lamp is essential in determining the presence of white blood cells or abnormal amounts of protein in the normally optically clear aqueous humor of the anterior chamber. The quantification of these abnormalities may help establish the diagnosis of uveitis and track disease activity and response to treatment [6] (Table 7.2).

Fig. 7.5 Intermediate uveitis with "snowballs" visible (yellow-white aggregates of inflammatory cells overlying the optic nerve and retinal vessels in the vitreous)

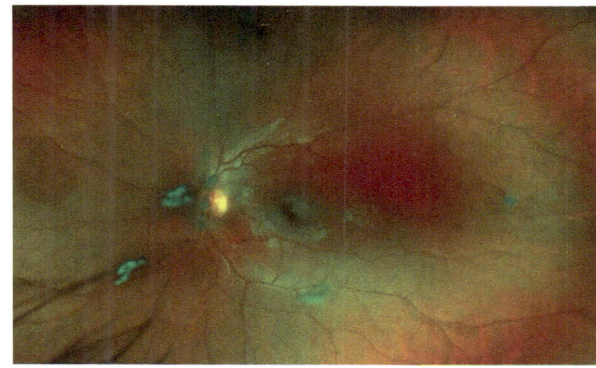

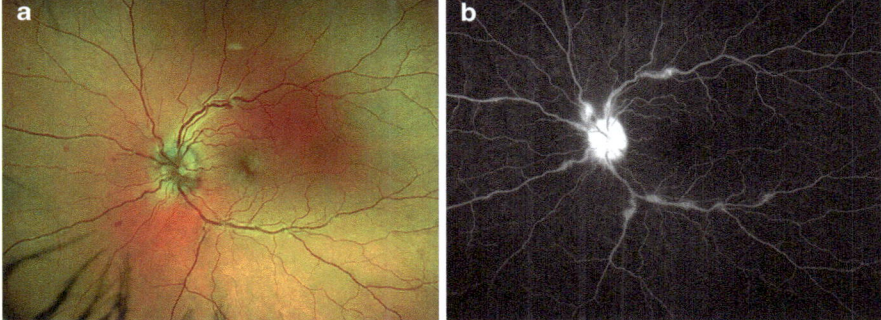

Fig. 7.6 (**a**) Sarcoidosis with granulomas, hemorrhage, and disc edema. (**b**) Fluorescein angiogram demonstrating inflammation of retinal veins (phlebitis) and the optic disc

Table 7.2 SUN working group grading scheme for anterior chamber cells and flare [6]

Grade of anterior chamber cells	Cells in field (field size = 1 mm × 1 mm slit beam)
0	<1
0.5+	1–5
1+	6–15
2+	16–25
3+	26–50
4+	>50
Grade of anterior chamber flare	Description
0	None
1+	Faint
2+	Moderate (iris and lens details clear)
3+	Marked (iris and lens details hazy)
4+	Intense (fibrin or plastic aqueous)

Table 7.3 Tailored evaluation for patients presenting with uveitis

Uveitic entity	Associated systemic conditions	Laboratory/imaging studies
Anterior uveitis *Pediatric*	JIA, TINU	ANA, CBC, urine beta-2 microglobulin, CMP
Adult	HLA B27-associated disease (inflammatory bowel disease, ankylosing spondylitis reactive arthritis, psoriatic arthritis) sarcoidosis, syphilis	HLA B27, CXR, TPPA
Intermediate uveitis	Multiple sclerosis, sarcoidosis, syphilis, malignancy, or masqueraders	CXR, CT chest (if CXR negative and suspicion is high), MRI brain, diagnostic vitrectomy (with flow cytometry, IL6/IL10, etc.)
Posterior uveitis/ panuveitis	Sarcoidosis, VKH, Behcet's, syphilis, VZV, HSV, CMV, toxoplasmosis	CXR, CT chest (if CXR negative and suspicion is high), anterior chamber or vitreous tap for PCR studies (viral or toxoplasmosis)

Laboratory Evaluation

Appropriate laboratory evaluation should be tailored to the most likely etiologies as indicated by patient demographics as well as features of the history and physical exam (Table 7.3).

Anterior uveitis
- Pediatric
- Juvenile Idiopathic Arthritis should be considered in cases of painless and chronic inflammation
- Anti-nuclear antibodies, ESR, rheumatoid factor, joint X-ray
- Tubulointerstitial nephritis and uveitis (TINU)
- Urinalysis, urine beta-2-microglobulin, creatinine, possible renal biopsy
- Adult

  - Variety of infectious and inflammatory causes are possible

    Test for syphilis, HLA-B27, ACE/lysozyme, chest CT

Intermediate uveitis
- Neurologic symptoms/multiple sclerosis: Brain MRI
- Ocular lymphoma: diagnostic vitrectomy
- ACE/lysozyme, lyme, chest CT, brain MRI

Posterior uveitis
- Fluorescein angiogram
- Toxoplasmosis, ACE/lysozyme, chest CT, QuantiFERON gold, VZV/HSV titers, syphilis

Treatment

Corticosteroids (topical or systemic) are the mainstay in the initial treatment of suspected non-infectious uveitis.

- Prednisolone acetate 1% eye drops frequently prescribed and well tolerated
    - Increased intraocular pressure/glaucoma possible with prolonged (>2 week) use of topical steroids
- Periocular steroid (sub-tenon injection) may be considered in severe and chronic cases when infection has been ruled out.

Cycloplegic medications may alleviate pain and photosensitivity by immobilizing the iris and ciliary body. These medications also help prevent the formation of posterior synechiae.

- Cyclopentolate has a moderate duration and is commonly prescribed
- Atropine is longer acting and may have anti-inflammatory properties by stabilizing the blood–aqueous barrier

Systemic steroid-sparing agents, such as methotrexate, are preferred in chronic cases requiring systemic immunosuppression. Biologic agents such as infliximab may also play a role [7].

Infectious etiologies require appropriate antimicrobial therapy. Bacterial infections may require intravitreal or systemic antibiotics while viral infections (acute retinal necrosis secondary to herpes simplex virus) require prompt treatment with systemic anti-viral medication.

- Topical and oral corticosteroids are often employed in these cases following 24–72 h of appropriate antimicrobial therapy

Complications

The inflammation associated with uveitis can result in several vision-threatening complications affecting the structures of the eye.

- Cornea—Band keratopathy
- Lens—Cataract
- Retina—Macular edema, retinal detachment
- Optic nerve—Glaucoma

Uncontrolled inflammation may ultimately result in phthisis bulbi and complete loss of vision. Early diagnosis and treatment often result in a favorable outcome, particularly in patients with anterior uveitis. Intermediate and posterior uveitis portend a more guarded prognosis and intractable inflammation may result in loss of vision despite therapy. Special care must be taken in patients with infectious uveitis as rapid progression to permanent visual disability is possible.

References

1. Gritz DC, Wong IG. Incidence and prevalence of uveitis in Northern California; the Northern California epidemiology of uveitis study. Ophthalmology. 2004;111(3):491–500.
2. Durrani OM, Meads CA, Murray PI. Uveitis: a potentially blinding disease. Ophthalmologica. 2004;218(4):223–36.
3. Durrani OM, Tehrani NN, Marr JE, Moradi P, Stavrou P, Murray PI. Degree, duration, and causes of visual loss in uveitis. Br J Ophthalmol. 2004;88(9):1159–62.
4. Sen HN, Davis J, Ucar D, Fox A, Chan CC, Goldstein DA. Gender disparities in ocular inflammatory disorders. Curr Eye Res. 2015;40(2):146–61.
5. Thorne JE, Suhler E, Skup M, Tari S, Macaulay D, Chao J, et al. Prevalence of noninfectious uveitis in the United States: a claims-based analysis. JAMA Ophthalmol. 2016;134(11):1237–45.
6. Standardization of Uveitis Nomenclature (SUN) Working Group. Standardization of uveitis nomenclature for reporting clinical data. Results of the first international workshop. Am J Ophthalmol. 2005;140(3):509–16.
7. Rosenbaum JT, Bodaghi B, Couto C, Zierhut M, Acharya N, Pavesio C, et al. New observations and emerging ideas in diagnosis and management of non-infectious uveitis: a review. Semin Arthritis Rheum. 2019;49(3):438–45.

Chapter 8
Pediatric Ophthalmology

Grace L. Su, Emily K. Tam, and Laura C. Huang

Introduction

Amblyopia is the most common cause of childhood-onset unilateral decreased vision in North America, with a prevalence of 2–4% [1, 2]. Routine ocular examination to evaluate refractive error and strabismic deviation is an important intervention to reduce the development of amblyopia. Treatment options for strabismus include glasses, penalization and/or patching therapy, and surgical intervention.

Amblyopia

- A unilateral or bilateral decrease of visual acuity not attributable to an ocular or visual pathway abnormality [3].

Pathophysiology

- Development of the visual pathway occurs during a critical period between zero and 2 years of age. During this time, the visual cortex is highly sensitive to environmental stimuli. The white matter of the visual pathways become increasingly

G. L. Su · E. K. Tam · L. C. Huang (✉)
Department of Ophthalmology, Seattle Children's Hospital and University of Washington, Seattle, WA, USA
e-mail: gracelsu@uw.edu; kayitam@uw.edu; lchuang1@uw.edu

© The Author(s), under exclusive license to Springer Nature Switzerland AG 2023
E. Li, C. Bacorn (eds.), *Ophthalmology Clerkship*, Contemporary Surgical Clerkships, https://doi.org/10.1007/978-3-031-27327-8_8

myelinated and synaptic connections continue to develop until approximately 10 years of age.
- Disruption of visual stimuli to this developing system can lead to amblyopia. This critical period of rapid development also allows for potential reversal of amblyopia with appropriate intervention.

Classification

- **Strabismic amblyopia:** Due to ocular misalignment. The visual cortex receives predominant input from the fixating eye, leading to amblyopia in the deviating eye.
- **Refractive amblyopia**: Images are not focused on the retina secondary to refractive error leading to decreased visual development.
    - Anisometropic: Due to dissimilar refractive errors between each eye. The eye with a higher refractive error receives a chronically defocused retinal image if uncorrected.
    - Bilateral ametropic: Bilateral decrease in vision due to large uncorrected refractive errors in both eyes.
    - Meridional: Chronically defocused images from high astigmatism.
- **Deprivational amblyopia**: Structural abnormality that occludes the visual axis. For example, congenital cataract (Fig. 8.1a), corneal changes (Fig. 8.1b), or eyelid obstruction from ptosis.
    - Although deprivational amblyopia is the least common, it is the most severe and difficult to treat.

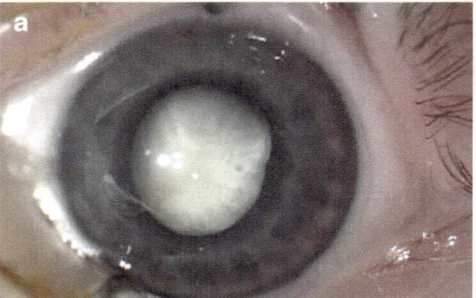 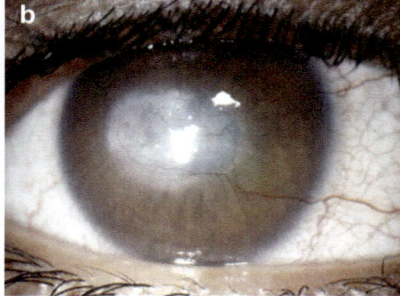

Fig. 8.1 (**a**) Dense cataract secondary to persistent fetal vasculature. (**b**) Dense axial corneal scar secondary to blepharokeratoconjunctivitis (*Republished with permission of Elsevier from Taylor and Hoyt's Pediatric Ophthalmology and Strabismus, Scott R. Lambert and Christopher J. Lyons, 5th ed. 2017; permission conveyed through Copyright Clearance Center, Inc.*)

Treatment

Treatment of amblyopia includes clearing the visual axis of obstruction, correcting the refractive error and any significant misalignment.

- **Refractive correction**
  - Cycloplegic spectacle correction is given to patients who are amblyopic or have strabismic misalignments that may increase the risk of developing amblyopia.
  - Refractive correction is first-line treatment initiated before other modalities such as patching or pharmacologic treatment [4].
- **Patching therapy**
  - Occlusion of the better seeing eye forces use of the amblyopic eye and drives visual development.
  - The amount of patching prescribed depends on the severity of amblyopia. Patients require frequent follow-up during treatment to assess response and prevent the development of "reverse amblyopia" (amblyopia of the formerly better seeing eye as a result of patching) [5, 6].
  - Severe amblyopia (visual acuity 20/125–20/400): 6 hours daily.
  - Moderate amblyopia (visual acuity 20/100 or better): 2 hours daily.
- **Penalization therapy**
  - Pharmacologic treatment involves administration of a cycloplegic agent to the non-amblyopic eye to blur vision and promote usage of the amblyopic eye.
  - Optical degradation treatment includes utilizing fogging or filters over glasses to blur vision in the non-amblyopic eye.
  - Both modalities can be effective in children and are useful for patients intolerant of patching.
- **Surgical therapy**
  - Deprivational amblyopia due to cataracts may be treated with cataract surgery. Visually significant cataracts are recommended to be removed by 6 weeks of age (if unilateral) or 8–10 weeks of age (if bilateral).
  - Surgical correction of strabismus may ultimately be required in cases of amblyogenic misalignment.

Strabismus

- Ocular misalignment
- May lead to amblyopia in the deviating eye

Esodeviations

Esodeviation refers to inward turning or convergence of the eyes and is the most common type of childhood strabismus [7]. Common etiologies of true esotropia include: congenital esotropia, accommodative esotropia, and non-accommodative esotropia (includes restrictive and innervational abnormalities of extraocular muscles).

- **Pseudoesotropia**
    - Patient has normal alignment without any deviation, but with appearance of esotropia due to a broad nasal bridge or prominent medial epicanthal folds.
    - Should be distinguished from true esotropia.
- **Congenital or infantile esotropia** (Fig. 8.2)
    - Occurs from birth to less than 6 months of age.
    - Risk factors: History of prematurity, neurologic and/or developmental problems.
    - Clinical features [8]: >30 prism diopters (PD) of deviation, low hyperopic refraction (+1.00 to +2.00 diopters), equal vision due to cross-fixation (the adducted eye is used to view the contralateral visual field) although amblyopia may occur if the child develops a fixation preference.
    - Treatment: Early strabismus surgery.

- **Accommodative esotropia** (Fig. 8.3a, b)
    - Occurs between 6 months and 7 years of age.
    - High uncorrected hyperopia leads to accommodation and convergence (as part of the near reflex triad).
    - Clinical features: Esotropia with moderate to high hyperopic correction that improves or resolves with spectacle correction.
    - Treatment: Full hyperopic refractive correction. Strabismus surgery usually reserved for any residual esodeviation not alleviated by glasses.

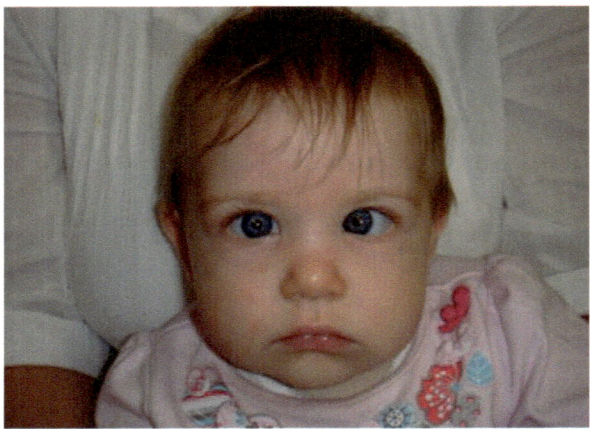

Fig. 8.2 Large angle infantile esotropia *(Republished with permission of Elsevier from Taylor and Hoyt's Pediatric Ophthalmology and Strabismus, Scott R. Lambert and Christopher J. Lyons, 5th ed. 2017; permission conveyed through Copyright Clearance Center, Inc.)*

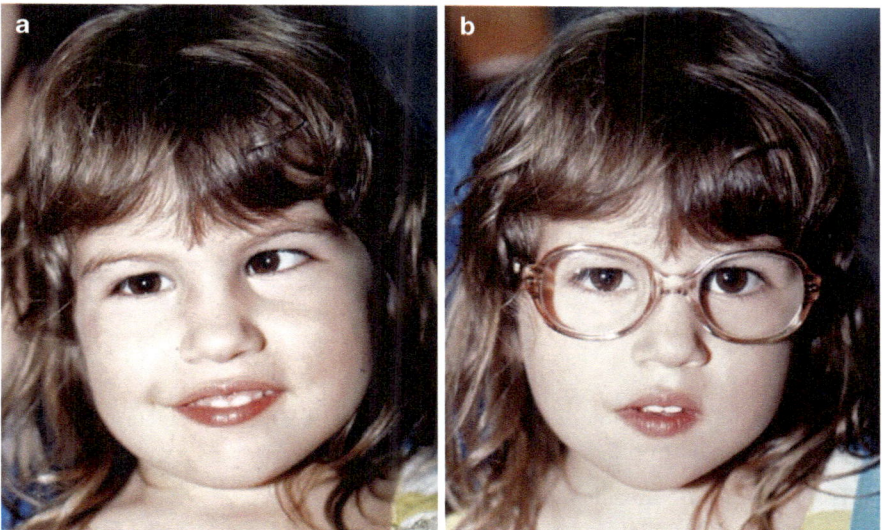

Fig. 8.3 (**a**) 3-year-old girl presented with a new onset of left esotropia (with strong fixation preference for the right eye). The deviation was 35 PD at near and distance fixation. Cycloplegic refraction was +4.25 in the right eye and +4.50 in the left eye. (**b**) The same girl, 4 weeks later, wearing her full hyperopic correction. She had a small left esotropia with fixation preference for her right eye. Part-time occlusion therapy of the right eye was begun *(Republished with permission of Elsevier from Taylor and Hoyt's Pediatric Ophthalmology and Strabismus, Scott R. Lambert and Christopher J. Lyons, 5th ed. 2017; permission conveyed through Copyright Clearance Center, Inc.)*

Exodeviations

Exodeviation refers to outward turning or divergence of the eyes. Common etiologies include intermittent exotropia as well as congenital exotropia.

- **Congenital exotropia**
  - Occurs from birth to less than 6 months of age.
  - Risk factors: Prematurity, perinatal morbidity, genetic anomalies.
  - Clinical features: Constant, large-angle exotropia.
  - Treatment: Early strabismus surgery. Consider neurology referral or brain imaging due to high risk of associated neurologic or craniofacial disorders in these patients [9].
- **Intermittent exotropia**
  - Most common type of manifest exodeviation.
  - Intermittent exodeviation that worsens with fatigue, stress, or illness. May decompensate into a constant exodeviation.
  - Occurs typically before 5 years of age.
  - Exodeviation control is divided into good, fair, and poor [10].

- Good: Manifests only after cover testing, and the patient resumes fusion immediately.
- Fair: Manifests after fusion is disrupted, and the patient resumes fusion only after blinking or refixating.
- Poor: Manifests spontaneously without disruption of fusion.
- Treatment: Treat any amblyopia and optimize spectacle correction.
- Strabismus surgery is recommended for poor control of exotropia, exotropia >50% of the time, and constant exotropia.

Vertical Deviations

A hyper- or hypo-deviation of an eye. Conventionally, vertical deviations are with respect to the hypertropic eye.

- **Inferior oblique muscle overaction**
  - Overelevation that is most prominent in adduction.
  - Commonly associated with infantile strabismus (esotropia or exotropia).
- **Fourth cranial nerve palsy**
  - Etiology: Congenital or acquired (trauma, diabetes, mass effect).
  - Clinical features: Hypertropia worsened in ipsilateral head tilt or contralateral gaze. These characteristics are the basis of the three-step test, also called the Parks–Bielschowsky test, that aids in the diagnosis of unilateral superior oblique muscle [11].
  - Patients often adopt a compensatory head tilt contralateral to the affected eye as this minimizes the vertical diplopia experienced.
  - Treatment: Strabismus surgery is indicated if there is a significant head tilt, large hypertropia in primary gaze, or presence of diplopia.
- **Dissociated vertical deviation (DVD)**
  - Associated with early disruption of binocular development in infantile strabismus.
  - Clinical features: The non-fixating eye intermittently drifts upward and outward, then moves down to fixate when the fellow eye is occluded.
  - The fellow eye does not refixate in the opposite direction, thus violates Hering's law.
  - Hering's law refers to the phenomena that the extraocular muscles receive equal innervation bilaterally so that the eyes move in concert with one another (maintain conjugate gaze).
  - Treatment: Treat any amblyopia and optimize spectacle correction.
  - Strabismus surgery is recommended for increasing size or frequency of a manifest hypertropia due to DVD.

Surgical Procedure for Strabismus

- While some ocular deviations may be managed with conservative management many require surgical realignment.
- Strabismus surgery can improve visual function, restore binocular fusion and stereopsis, relieve asthenopia (eye strain), improve appearance, and expand the binocular visual field.
- Strabismus surgery in children is performed under general anesthesia.
- Ocular alignment may be achieved by weakening the action of muscles responsible for the eye deviation or strengthening the action of muscles that oppose the deviation. In order to correct large deviations, multiple muscles may be required.

Types of Surgical Procedures

Weakening Procedures

- Recession: A muscle is detached from its insertion on the globe and reattached to the sclera in a more posterior position closer to its origin (Fig. 8.4).
- Myotomy: Cutting partial thickness across a muscle (used for inferior oblique muscle).
- Myectomy: Excising a portion of the muscle for complete removal (used for inferior oblique muscle).
- Tenotomy: Cutting partial thickness across a tendon (used for superior oblique muscle).

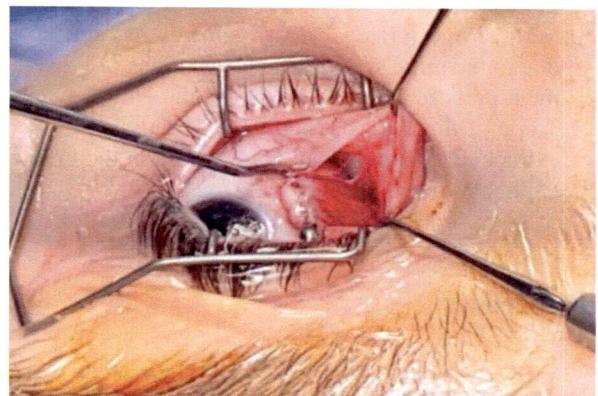

Fig. 8.4 The medial rectus of the left eye is isolated during surgery in preparation for a medial rectus recession to treat an esotropia

Strengthening Procedures

- Resection: A segment of muscle is removed, and its insertion is reattached at its original site. This shortens the muscle belly and increases its action.
- Plication: A segment of muscle is folded over and sutured to shorten the muscle without disrupting the insertion site.

Other Procedures

- Transposition: A muscle is disinserted and reattached to the sclera near the insertion of a paretic muscle to improve motility in this direction.

Examples

- Esotropia occurs when the eyes are directed medially. This may be corrected in a number of ways depending on surgeon preference and the specific details of the esodeviation.
  - Bilateral medial rectus recession: The medial recti of the left and right eye are recessed to weaken the adducting forces on both eyes.
  - Unilateral recess/resect: The non-fixating eye is typically selected for surgery. The medial rectus is recessed and the lateral rectus is resected in order to rotate the eye laterally and improve alignment.
- Exotropia may be treated analogously with bilateral lateral recti recessions or a unilateral medial rectus resection and lateral rectus recession.
- In small angle deviations, surgery on single muscles may be possible, such as a unilateral medial rectus recession in the treatment of a small esotropia.
- Vertical and torsional misalignments require more complex surgical planning due to the more significant contributions of the oblique muscles to ocular alignment in these cases. Treatment of these more complex procedures is beyond the scope of this text, but additional discussion of the anatomy and actions of the extraocular muscles may be reviewed in the Overview of Anatomy and Neuro-Ophthalmology chapters.

References

1. McKean-Cowdin R, Cotter SA, Tarczy-Hornoch K, Wen G, Kim J, Borchert M, Varma R, Multi-Ethnic Pediatric Eye Disease Study Group. Prevalence of amblyopia or strabismus in Asian and non-Hispanic white preschool children: multi-ethnic pediatric eye disease study. Ophthalmology. 2013;120(10):2117–24.
2. Multi-ethnic Pediatric Eye Disease Study Group. Prevalence of amblyopia and strabismus in African American and Hispanic children ages 6–72 months the multi-ethnic pediatric eye disease study. Ophthalmology. 2008;115(7):1229–36.

3. Blair K, Cibis G, Gulani AC. Amblyopia. Treasure Island (FL): StatPearls Publishing; 2022.
4. Writing Committee for the Pediatric Eye Disease Investigator Group, Cotter SA, Foster NC, Holmes JM, Melia BM, Wallace DK, Repka MX, Tamkins SM, Kraker RT, Beck RW, Hoover DL, Crouch ER 3rd, Miller AM, Morse CL, Suh DW. Optical treatment of strabismic and combined strabismic-anisometropic amblyopia. Ophthalmology. 2012;119(1):150–8.
5. Repka MX, Beck RW, Holmes JM, Birch EE, Chandler DL, Cotter SA, Hertle RW, Kraker RT, Moke PS, Quinn GE, Scheiman MM, Pediatric Eye Disease Investigator Group. A randomized trial of patching regimens for treatment of moderate amblyopia in children. Arch Ophthalmol. 2003;121(5):603–11.
6. Holmes JM, Kraker RT, Beck RW, Birch EE, Cotter SA, Everett DF, Hertle RW, Quinn GE, Repka MX, Scheiman MM, Wallace DK, Pediatric Eye Disease Investigator Group. A randomized trial of prescribed patching regimens for treatment of severe amblyopia in children. Ophthalmology. 2003;110(11):2075–87.
7. Repka MX, Yu F, Coleman A. Strabismus among aged fee-for-service Medicare beneficiaries. J AAPOS. 2012;16(6):495–500.
8. Pediatric Eye Disease Investigator Group. The clinical spectrum of early-onset esotropia: experience of the congenital Esotropia observational study. Am J Ophthalmol. 2002;133(1):102–8.
9. Lueder GT, Galli M. Infantile exotropia and developmental delay. J Pediatr Ophthalmol Strabismus. 2018;55(4):225–8.
10. Burian HM. Exodeviations: their classification, diagnosis and treatment. Am J Ophthalmol. 1966;62(6):1161–6.
11. Bielschowsky A. Lecture on motor anomalies of the eyes: II. Paralysis of individual eye muscles. Arch Ophthalmol. 1935;13:33–59.

Chapter 9
Neuro-Ophthalmology

Alberto Distefano, Lindsay Rothfield, and Jia Xu

Visual Pathway

The perception of light and visual stimuli is made possible by the transmission of electrochemical impulses from the retina to the visual cortex along the following structures (Fig. 9.1). An understanding of the anatomy of these pathways allows for the localization of lesions causing visual field defects.

Retina

- The retinal nerve fibers are made up of the axons originating from the ganglion cells of the inner retina.
- Retinal nerve fibers originating nasally carry visual information from the temporal visual field while temporally originating fibers carry information from the nasal visual field.

A. Distefano (✉)
Department of Ophthalmology, Boston University School of Medicine, Boston, MA, USA

Department of Ophthalmology, Icahn School of Medicine at Mount Sinai, New York, NY, USA
e-mail: alberto.distefano@mssm.edu

L. Rothfield · J. Xu
Department of Ophthalmology, Boston University School of Medicine, Boston, MA, USA
e-mail: lindsay.rothfield@bmc.org; jia.xu@bmc.org

E. Li, C. Bacorn (eds.), *Ophthalmology Clerkship*, Contemporary Surgical Clerkships, https://doi.org/10.1007/978-3-031-27327-8_9

123

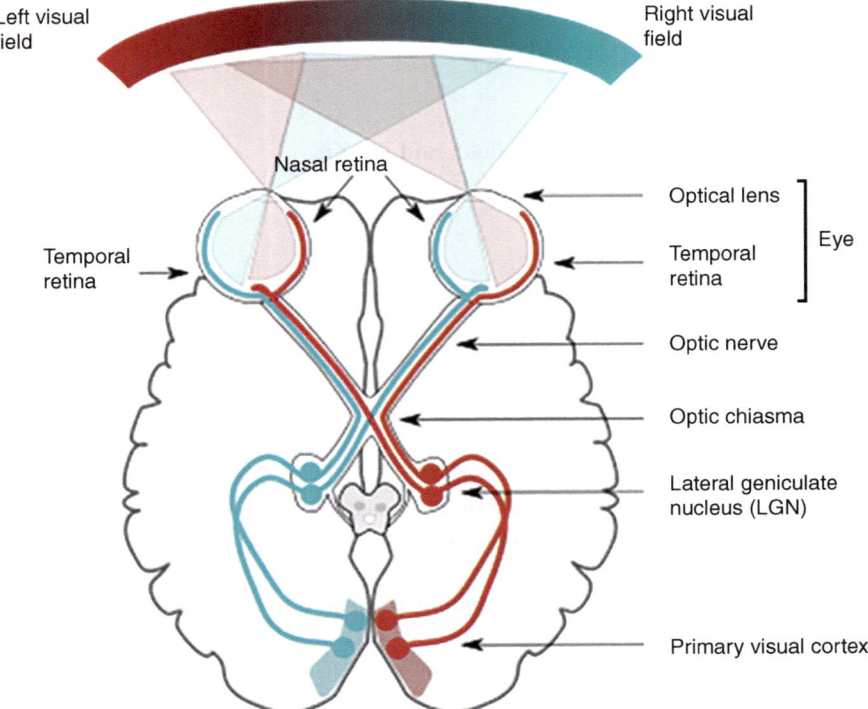

Fig. 9.1 Anatomic arrangement of the visual pathway demonstrating the decussation of the left and right visual fields

Optic Nerve

- Each optic nerve represents a collection of 770,000 to 1.7 million nerve fibers which exit the posterior globe to pass through the orbit and into the cranium [1, 2].
- The optic nerve is vulnerable to ischemic and toxic insults (optic **neuropathy**) as well as inflammatory processes (optic **neuritis**).

Optic Chiasm

- The right and left optic nerves join at the chiasm, which is located within the cranium superior to the sella turcica, inferior to the pituitary gland, and anterior to the hypothalamus and third ventricle.

  - Compression of the optic chiasm classically causes temporal visual field loss in both eyes (**bitemporal hemianopia**).

- Nasal fibers from each optic nerve decussate at the chiasm to join the contralateral nerve's temporal fibers and form left and right **optic tracts**.

  - Unilateral lesions of the visual pathway posterior to the optic chiasm will result in symmetric bilateral (**homonymous**) visual field defects [1, 2].

Optic Tract

- Each optic tract is a conduit of axons originating from the ipsilateral temporal retina and contralateral nasal retina.

  - As a result of this anatomic arrangement, the right optic tract carries fibers responsible for the left visual field and vice versa.
  - A lesion of the right optic tract results in the loss of perception of the left visual field in both eyes (**homonymous hemianopia**).

- A subset of axons responsible for the afferent pupillary response diverge from the visual pathway by exiting the optic tract and traveling to the pretectal nucleus and Edinger–Westphal nucleus.
- Axons of the optic tract synapse in the lateral geniculate nucleus in the midbrain [1, 2].

Optic Radiation

- Axons from the cell bodies of the lateral geniculate nucleus travel to the occipital lobe and visual cortex, forming the optic radiations.
- Each optic radiation is divided into inferior (travels through the temporal lobe) and superior divisions (travels through the parietal lobe).

  - A lesion of the right superior optic radiation causes loss of the left inferior quadrant of vision in both eyes (inferior **quadrantanopia**) while a lesion of the left inferior optic radiation will result in a right superior quadrantanopia in both eyes [1, 2].

Visual Cortex

- The visual cortex is a region of the occipital lobe responsible for the initial processing of visual information. Information is conveyed from the primary visual cortex to multiple other cortical regions for higher level processing of visual stimuli.

  - Lesions of the visual cortex may result in central scotomas or quadrantanopias [1, 2].

Afferent Pupillary Pathway

The pupil constricts and dilates in response to increasing or decreasing levels of retinal illumination, respectively. This response is independent of the conscious perception of light and the responsible pathway is largely anatomically distinct from the previously described visual pathway. Due to the decussations along this pathway, the normal pupillary responses are **consensual** (dilate or constrict simultaneously with unilateral exposure to light).

- Afferent pupillary pathway: retina → optic nerve → optic chiasm → optic tract → pretectal nuclei (synapse) → Edinger–Westphal nuclei (synapse) (Fig. 9.2).

  - This pathway decussates twice at the (1) optic chiasm and (2) at the pretectal nucleus [1, 2].

- A **relative afferent pupillary defect** (rAPD) refers to the finding of a stronger response to light (more constriction) with unilateral illumination of one eye compared to unilateral illumination of the contralateral eye. A right rAPD indicates that the right and left pupils constrict to a lesser degree when light is shone into the right eye than when light is shone into the left eye.

  - The presence of an rAPD most commonly indicates pathology of the optic nerve and is a very useful clinical test for differentiating optic nerve-related vision loss from other causes.

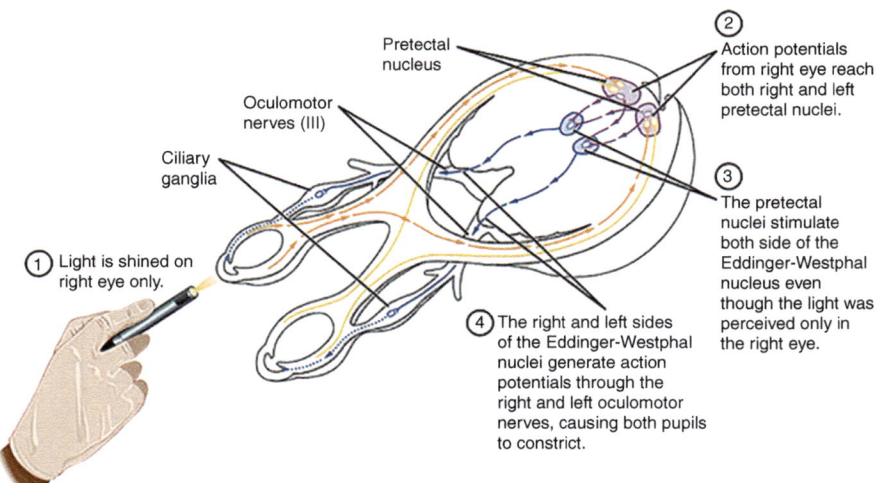

Fig. 9.2 Anatomy of the afferent pupillary response. Unilateral light stimuli trigger bilateral pupillary constriction due decussation at the pretectal nuclei triggering bilateral parasympathetic neurons of the Edinger–Westphal nucleus

Efferent Pupillary Pathway

Pupil size is dictated by the sympathetically innervated iris dilator and parasympathetically innervated iris sphincter muscles. Activation of these muscles is normally dictated by the level of illumination of the retina and transmission along the afferent pupillary pathway. Systemic and topical medications can bypass the efferent pupillary pathways to affect pupil size independent of ambient light levels.

Parasympathetic Pathway

- The parasympathetic pathway is responsible for iris constriction in response to increased illumination. Functionally, it represents a continuation of the afferent pupillary pathway.
- Parasympathetic pathway: Edinger–Westphal nucleus → oculomotor nerve → ciliary ganglion (synapse) → short ciliary nerve → iris sphincter muscle (Fig. 9.2) [1, 2]

Sympathetic Pathway

- The sympathetic pathway is responsible for iris dilation in response to increased adrenergic tone ("fight or flight"), distinct from the visual and afferent pupillary pathways.
- The sympathetic pathway is an uncrossed (non-decussating) three-neuron pathway. Lesions at any level of the pathway can result in anisocoria and may be localized with careful clinical testing (Fig. 9.3).

  - First-order neurons travel from cell bodies in the hypothalamus to synapse at the ciliospinal center of Budge (C8–T2 spinal levels).
  - Second-order neurons travel from the ciliospinal center of Budge along the apex of the lung to synapse at the superior cervical ganglion at the bifurcation of the carotid artery.
  - Third-order neurons (aka "post-ganglionic" neurons) travel from the superior cervical ganglion through the cavernous sinus and into the orbit with the long ciliary nerves to innervate the iris dilator muscle.

    In addition to the iris dilator muscle, these sympathetic fibers also innervate **Muller's** muscle of the upper eyelid, accounting for two of the three classic findings of **Horner's syndrome** (ipsilateral miosis and ptosis; other fibers are responsible for the finding of anhidrosis) [1, 2].

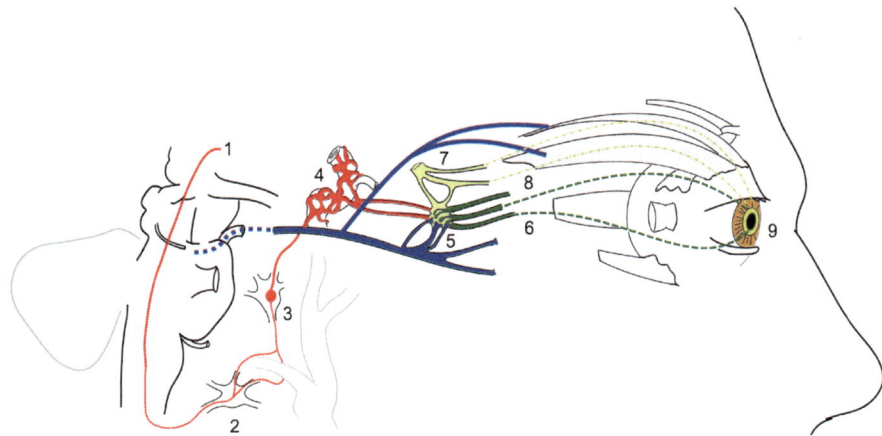

Fig. 9.3 Illustration of the course of the first-, second-, and third-order neurons of the sympathetic pathway which runs from the hypothalamus to the ipsilateral pupil

Anisocoria

Anisocoria is a common clinical presentation with a wide variety of underlying etiologies. These etiologies range from benign and physiologic to imminently life-threatening, making interpretation of pupillary exam findings extremely important.

- Anisocoria is defined as a difference in pupil size and is considered pathologic when greater than 1 mm.
- Without additional information, it cannot be determined whether the larger (**mydriatic**) pupil or the smaller (**miotic**) pupil is abnormal. Careful examination of both pupils' response to light, and in some cases pharmacologic testing, can determine which side is pathologic as well as the likely underlying etiology (Fig. 9.4)
  - Anisocoria that is greater in bright light than in dim light indicates a failure in the mydriatic pupil to constrict and pathology of the parasympathetic pathway.
  - Anisocoria that is greater in dim light than in bright light indicates a failure in the miotic pupil to dilate and pathology of the sympathetic pathway [3].

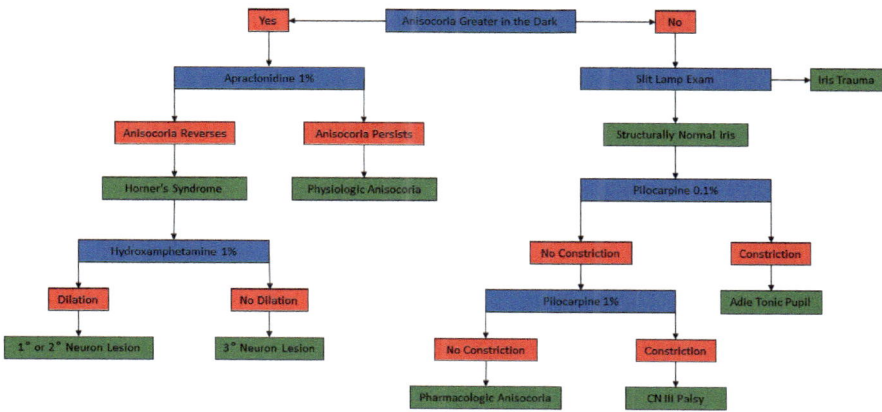

Fig. 9.4 Algorithm for the evaluation of anisocoria and several clinically important diagnostic considerations

Motor Pathway

Cranial Nerve III (Oculomotor)

Cranial nerve III (CN III) is a complex, multi-functioned, nerve that is responsible for the motor function of several muscles within and surrounding the globe. The details of the nuclei of cranial nerve III and the nerve's sub-branching are beyond the scope of this text, but the remainder of this discussion will highlight the nerve's main functions and their clinical significance.

- CN III originates from the oculomotor nucleus in the midbrain with parasympathetic contributions from the Edinger–Westphal nucleus.

  - Its motor axons are arranged centrally within the nerve while parasympathetic axons travel peripherally.

CN III innervates the following muscles
- Superior Rectus: Elevation of the globe
- Inferior Rectus: Depression of the globe
- Medial Rectus: Adduction of the globe
- Inferior Oblique: **Excyclotorsion** (12 o'clock position of the globe is rotated temporally when viewed along the anterior–posterior axis) of the globe.
- Levator Palpebrae: Elevation of the superior eyelid.
- Iris Sphincter Muscle: Constriction of the pupil; previously discussed in the afferent pupillary pathway [4].

Cranial Nerve III Palsy

- Complete loss of function (complete CN III palsy) results in ipsilateral:
  - "Down and Out" eye position (eye is depressed and abducted due to residual function of the lateral rectus and superior oblique).
  - Ptosis.
  - Mydriasis.
- Partial CN III palsies may involve any of the functions of the nerve, but a key differentiator is pupillary function.
  - Pupil-involving (affected pupil is dilated).

    True potentially life-threatening emergency.
    Pathology of the peripherally oriented parasympathetic fibers of CN III suggests a compressive lesion, such as an aneurysm of the posterior communicating artery.
    Requires emergent evaluation with neuro-imaging and CT or MR angiography.
  - Pupil-sparing.

    Most commonly caused by a microvascular ischemic insult to CN III, especially in older adults with vascular risk factors.
    Rarely, a compressive lesion can present as a pupil-sparing CN III palsy.
    Requires close follow-up but in many cases resolves without intervention.
- Etiology
  - Ischemia (most commonly from diabetes or hypertension).
  - Trauma.
  - Mass effect (tumors, aneurysms, or hemorrhage).
  - Congenital.
  - Inflammatory.
  - Idiopathic [5].

Cranial Nerve IV (Trochlear)

Cranial nerve IV (CN IV) is a small and delicate nerve with a long intracranial course, which pre-disposes it to trauma.

- Originates from its nucleus in the midbrain before nerve fibers decussate and exit the brainstem dorsally.
- It enters the cavernous sinus and travels laterally until entering the orbit through the superior orbital fissure (outside and superior to the annulus of Zinn) to innervate the superior oblique muscle.

- Its sole function is the innervation of the superior oblique muscle, which primarily serves to **incyclotort** the globe (lesser actions are depression and abduction) [6].

Cranial Nerve IV Palsy

- Generally, CN IV palsy presents with vertical diplopia and examination may demonstrate a hypertropia of the affected eye.
    - Diplopia is classically worse in contralateral gaze or ipsilateral head tilt.
- Etiology
    - Congenital

        May be distinguished from an acute palsy by photographs demonstrating a chronic head tilt or the presence of large vertical fusional amplitudes on examination.

    - Ischemia
    - Trauma

        Frequently can present with bilateral involvement

    - Mass effect
    - Idiopathic
- Diagnosis
    - Ipsilateral hypertropia that worsens with contralateral gaze and ipsilateral head tilt.
    - Large vertical fusional amplitudes.
    - Hypertension and diabetes studies to assess microvascular risk factors.
    - Neuro-imaging with brain MRI if associated with other cranial nerve or neurologic findings.
- Treatment.
    - Treat the underlying disorder.
    - Symptomatic relief of diplopia by using occlusion patch or prism glasses.
    - Consider strabismus surgery if persistent and stable in measurements after 6 months [3, 6].

Superior Oblique Myokymia

- Spasm of the superior oblique muscle of unknown etiology
- Can be associated with dry eyes, stress, caffeine, alcohol, and fatigue
- Can occasionally cause superior oblique weakness
    - Clinical diagnosis [3]

Cranial Nerve VI (Abducens)

Cranial nerve VI has the second longest intracranial course and innervates the ipsilateral lateral rectus muscle, which abducts the eye. It also contributes to the function of the contralateral medial rectus muscle via the medial longitudinal fasciculus (MLF).

- CN VI originates from the dorsal caudal pons and exits the brainstem at the pontomedullary junction before traversing the intracranial space to enter the cavernous sinus.

  - Axons from the CN VI nucleus decussate and trigger the contralateral CN III nucleus to coordinate simultaneous contraction of the lateral rectus muscle with the medial rectus muscle of the opposite eye to facilitate conjugate lateral gaze (e.g., right eye abduction occurs with simultaneous left eye adduction) [7].

Cranial Nerve VI Palsy

- Presents with horizontal diplopia with an abduction deficit in the effected eye.
- Etiology

  - Ischemia

    Most common cause.
    Secondary to microvascular disease (e.g., diabetes, hypertension).
    Nerve function typically recovers within 6 months.

  - Congenital.
  - Trauma.
  - Compression.
  - Elevated intracranial pressure.
  - Infection.
  - Demyelinating syndromes.
  - Idiopathic.

- Diagnosis.

  - Esotropia worse on abduction of the involved eye.
  - Obtain blood pressure and HbA1c to assess for microvascular risk factors.
  - Neuro-imaging with brain MRI if associated with other cranial nerve or neurologic findings.

    Children may require a full work-up even in the absence of additional findings given a higher probability of intracranial malignancy in the setting of a new adduction deficit.

- Treatment.
    - Treat the underlying disorder.
    - Symptomatic relief of diplopia by using occlusion patch or prisms.
    - Can consider strabismus surgery if persistent and stable in measurements after 6 months [3, 7].

Internuclear Ophthalmoplegia

- Clinical syndrome consisting of impaired ipsilateral adduction with contralateral nystagmus with abduction.
    - Caused by injury to the **medial longitudinal fasciculus,** which transmits information from the CN VI nucleus to the contralateral CN III nucleus.
    - Often seen in demyelinating disease such as multiple sclerosis [8].

Cavernous Sinus Syndrome

The cavernous sinus is a dural venous sinus on either side of the pituitary gland that contains many important structures and is the key site of venous drainage from the orbit. Disease of the cavernous sinus is critical to recognize as it may be vision or life-threatening.

- Anatomy
    - Each sinus rests on either side of the sphenoid bone in close proximity to the temporal lobe.
    - Contains:

        Motor Nerves: CN III, CN IV, CN VI.
        Sensory Nerves: V1, V2.
        Carotid Artery.
        Third order sympathetic nerves.

    - Notably, the optic nerve (CN II) does not travel through the cavernous sinus.
- Clinical findings indicating pathology
    - Total or partial ophthalmoplegia involving palsies of CN III, CN IV, and CN VI.
    - Facial sensory loss due to involvement of CN V1 and CN V2.
    - Horner syndrome due to involvement of the sympathetic plexus.
    - Proptosis and chemosis due to impaired venous drainage.

- Etiology.
  - Arterio-Venous (AV) fistula.

    Aberrant communication between blood flow in the carotid artery and the surrounding venous plexus causing increased venous pressure and impaired orbital drainage.

  - Cavernous sinus thrombosis.
  - Infection.
  - Tumor.
- Diagnosis.
  - Complete blood count (CBC), blood cultures.
  - Neuro-imaging with MRI/magnetic resonance venogram (MRV).
- Treatment.
  - Dependent on etiology.

    AV fistulas may require urgent neurosurgical intervention. Infections require broad spectrum antibiotics [2, 3].

Optic Disc Edema

Optic disc edema is a vision-threatening process characterized by swelling of the optic nerve head ("disc"). Causes are diverse, and a careful history and physical exam are necessary to determine the best next steps.

- Clinical findings
  - Symptoms: Headache, nausea, vomiting, **transient visual obscuration** (visual black out lasting seconds), pain with eye movement.
  - Signs: Decreased visual acuity, decreased color vision, rAPD, enlarged blind spot.
- Exam findings: Hyperemia of optic nerve head, disc hemorrhages, opacification of retinal nerve fiber layer, and obscuration of retinal vessels (Fig. 9.5).
- Etiology
  - Increased intracranial pressure (true **papilledema**).
  - Drusen/anatomic variation (**pseudopapilledema**).
  - Optic neuritis.

    Multiple sclerosis, neuromyelitis optica, syphilis, bartonella, Lyme disease, tuberculosis.

Fig. 9.5 Fundus photograph demonstrating severe disc edema (Frisen grade 5) with extensive surrounding hemorrhage

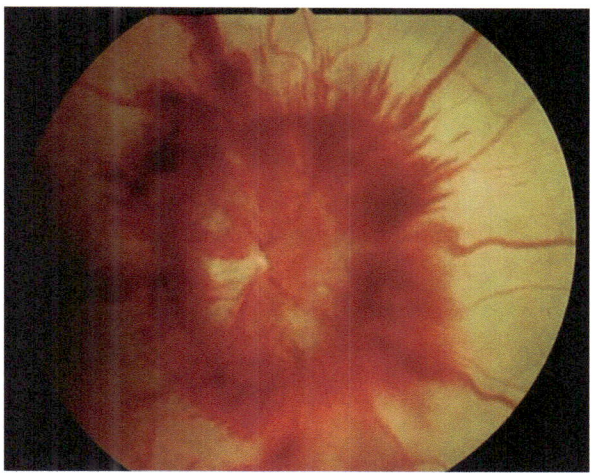

- Ischemic optic neuropathy.

  Arteritic (giant cell arteritis).
  Non-arteritic—vasculopathy common in patients with ischemic risk factors (e.g., smoking, hypertension, diabetes) and patients with a "disc at risk" (cup-to-disc ratio <0.1).

- Mechanical compression.
- Hereditary (Leber hereditary optic neuropathy).
- Toxic or nutritional optic neuropathy.

• Diagnosis

- Ophthalmic testing: Fundus photographs, automated visual field testing, optical coherence tomography (OCT).
- Laboratory testing: CBC, erythrocyte sedimentation rate (ESR)/c-reactive protein (CRP), anti-myelin oligodendrocyte glycoprotein (MOG) antibodies, aquaporin-4 antibodies, infectious serologies.
- Imaging:

  MRI brain and orbit with and without contrast with fat suppression.
  Fat suppression allows for evaluation of the intra-orbital portion of the optic nerve, which is otherwise masked by the strong signal from orbital fat.

- Procedures:

  Consider lumbar puncture in appropriate scenarios after obtaining neuro-imaging.
  Consider temporal artery biopsy if giant cell arteritis is suspected.

- Treatment

Increased intracranial pressure: Weight loss, acetazolamide, topiramate, optic nerve sheath fenestration, venous sinus stenting, ventriculoperitoneal shunting.
Optic neuritis: Intravenous steroids.

• Oral steroids are contraindicated. Steroid treatment hastens recovery but does not improve outcomes or prevent recurrence.

Giant cell arteritis: High dose oral steroids, tocilizumab.
Vasculopathy: Optimize blood pressure and cholesterol management, avoid sildenafil [9].

References

1. Armstrong RA, Cubbidge RC. Chapter 1: The eye and vision: an overview. In: Preedy VR, Watson RR, editors. Handbook of nutrition, diet, and the eye. 2nd ed. Cambridge: Academic Press; 2019. p. 3–14.
2. Bhatti MT, Biousse V, Bose S, Danesh-Meyer HV, Falardeau J, Levin LA, Phillips PH, Williams ZR. Section 5: Neuro-ophthalmology. In: 2018–2019 BCSC basic and clinical science course. San Francisco: American Academy of Ophthalmology; 2018.
3. Ehlers JP, Shah C, Fenton G, Hoskins E, Shelsta H. The Wills eye manual: office and emergency room diagnosis and treatment of eye diseases. 5th ed. Baltimore: Lippincott Williams & Wilkins; 2008.
4. Joyce C, Le PH, Peterson DC. Neuroanatomy, cranial nerve 3 (oculomotor). Treasure Island (FL): StatPearls Publishing; 2022.
5. Graham C, Mohseni M. Abducens nerve palsy. Treasure Island (FL): StatPearls Publishing; 2022.
6. Kim SY, Motlagh M, Naqvi IA. Neuroanatomy, cranial nerve 4 (trochlear). Treasure Island (FL): StatPearls Publishing; 2022.
7. Nguyen V, Reddy V, Varacallo M. Neuroanatomy, cranial nerve 6 (abducens). Treasure Island (FL): StatPearls Publishing; 2022.
8. Virgo JD, Plant GT. Internuclear ophthalmoplegia. Pract Neurol. 2017;17(2):149–53.
9. Rigi M, Almarzouqi SJ, Morgan ML, Lee AG. Papilledema: epidemiology, etiology, and clinical management. Eye Brain. 2015;7:47–57.

Chapter 10
On Call Issues

N. Maxwell Scoville, Alexandra Van Brummen, Samuel Kushner-Lenhoff, and Nicole R. Mattson

Trauma

Trauma to the orbital and ocular structures is common in patients presenting with facial trauma [1]. These traumatic injuries can be threatening to vision, and thus require careful evaluation to maximize the chance of vision preservation or recovery.

History Taking

- These patients may present in a variety of states, ranging from conscious and fully aware to intubated and sedated.
- Obtain a detailed history of the trauma, including timing and mechanism of injury.
- Talk to the patient, family members, friends, and other potential witnesses, as well as reviewing electronic and physical records.
- A thorough history will then inform the evaluation, including the focus of the physical exam and subsequent work-up. For instance, if the history was significant for a high velocity projectile injury consideration should be given to possible penetration of the orbit, globe, or skull.

N. M. Scoville (✉)
Department of Ophthalmology, University of Washington, Seattle, WA, USA

Department of Ophthalmology, The Ohio State University, Columbus, OH, USA

A. Van Brummen · S. Kushner-Lenhoff · N. R. Mattson
Department of Ophthalmology, University of Washington, Seattle, WA, USA
e-mail: avanbrum@uw.edu; kushnerl@uw.edu; nmattson@uw.edu

© The Author(s), under exclusive license to Springer Nature Switzerland AG 2023
E. Li, C. Bacorn (eds.), *Ophthalmology Clerkship*, Contemporary Surgical Clerkships, https://doi.org/10.1007/978-3-031-27327-8_10

Physical Exam

- Begin with an evaluation of the external structures, such as the eyelids and peri-orbital soft tissue, and then proceed inwards towards the ocular structures, such as the conjunctiva, sclera, iris, and ocular media.
- If periorbital tissue is swollen such that it becomes difficult to examine the eye itself, use Desmarres retractors to move the eyelids and expose the globe. To do this, hook an adequately sized retractor under each eyelid and retract such that the main direction of force is perpendicular to a coronal plane through the eye—this will avoid undue pressure to the globe itself. Once the eye is exposed, proceed with a careful evaluation of the ocular structures.

Ancillary Tests [2]

- Most patients with significant facial trauma deserve a dedicated computed tomography (CT) scan.
  - Ensure that CT scans include thin slices (0.5–1 mm) of the orbit to better characterize fracture patterns or identify small foreign objects.
- Ultrasound can also be helpful in evaluating the globe and identify things like retinal detachments or vitreous hemorrhage but should only be pursued after first ruling out an open globe injury.

Selected Diagnoses [2–5]

- **Orbital fractures:** The bony orbit is divided into the orbital roof, floor, lateral wall, and medial wall. Each section is composed of more than one bone—any of which can be fractured during an injury. Apart from fractures of the bony orbit, other orbital tissues can be damaged in injuries, including extraocular muscles, nerves, and blood vessels. Patients with orbital fractures commonly endorse pain and have significant periorbital swelling but may otherwise have a normal ophthalmologic evaluation. If uncomplicated, orbital fractures can be managed conservatively, including icing to reduce swelling and sinus precautions to prevent expansion of the orbital fracture. Surgical intervention may be indicated if patient exhibits signs of complications, noted below.
  - **Entrapped extraocular muscle:** Suspect if the patient exhibits limitation in movement of the eye in the direction opposite of the involved muscle (e.g., limitation in supraduction if the inferior rectus muscle is entrapped). Patients may also endorse double vision, severe pain with eye movement, and even nausea and bradycardia with eye movement due to the oculocardiac reflex.

- *Avulsed extraocular muscle:* Suspect if the patient exhibits limitation in movement of the eye in the direction of the involved muscle (e.g., limitation in adduction if medial rectus is avulsed).
- *Traumatic optic neuropathy:* Suspect if the patient exhibits vision loss associated with a relative afferent pupillary defect.
- *Orbital compartment syndrome:* This is caused by retrobulbar pathology (usually hemorrhage) that causes rise in pressure within the orbit which can lead to rapid vision loss due to optic nerve ischemia. Suspect if the CT reveals retrobulbar pathology, the eye appears proptotic, and the intraocular pressure is elevated. In this scenario, performing a lateral canthotomy and inferior cantholysis may alleviate the pressure. In extreme cases, superior cantholysis may also be necessary.

• *Eyelid lacerations:* Take note of length, depth, presence of contamination, involvement of critical eyelid structures such as the eyelid margin or the canalicular system (if medial to the lacrimal puncta), or violation of the orbital septum (suspect if there is prolapsed orbital fat). Involvement of the canalicular system may be confirmed by gently passing a probe into the canaliculus and observing exposed metal at the site of injury. Prior to repair cleanse the wound with normal saline irrigation and betadine. Many lacerations can be repaired at the bedside, but if complex they may need to be repaired in the operating room. After repair, the patient should use topical ointment containing antibiotics and keep the area clean while healing occurs. Prophylactic oral antibiotics are usually not indicated but may be prescribed if the wound was contaminated or the lacerations extended into the orbit.

- *Simple and superficial lacerations:* Reapproximate with tissue glue or with simple interrupted or running absorbable sutures.
- *Deep lacerations:* Place deep sutures to approximate deeper tissues (avoid incorporating the orbital septum in the suture if it has been violated) prior to closure of the skin as above.
- *Margin-involving lacerations:* The margin should be reapproximated with one or two vertical mattress sutures prior to closure of deep and superficial tissue layers as above.
- *Canalicular-involving lacerations:* Stents may need to be placed prior to laceration repair to maintain patency of the canalicular system as healing takes place.

• *Open globe injuries:* Defined as an injury in which the integrity of the wall of the eye (scleral and/or cornea) has been violated. Suspect if the globe appears deflated, if it is difficult to identify the ocular structures, or if there is significant hemorrhage. A specific sign associated with open globe injuries is the Seidel sign. The presence of aqueous humor egress from the eye is a positive Seidel sign. This is visualized under a cobalt-blue light after a fluorescein strip is applied to the eye in the area of the suspected laceration (Fig. 10.1). Imaging with CT can reveal irregular globe contour or intraocular hemorrhage. If suspicious of an open globe injury, surgical exploration and repair within 24 h is indicated. Ensure the patient's tetanus status is up to date, secure a rigid eye shield over the eye

Fig. 10.1 Seidel sign: after a fluorescein strip is touched to the cornea, aqueous leaks from the anterior chamber, visualized as a border of fluorescein with central clearing. (© 2022 American Academy of Ophthalmology)

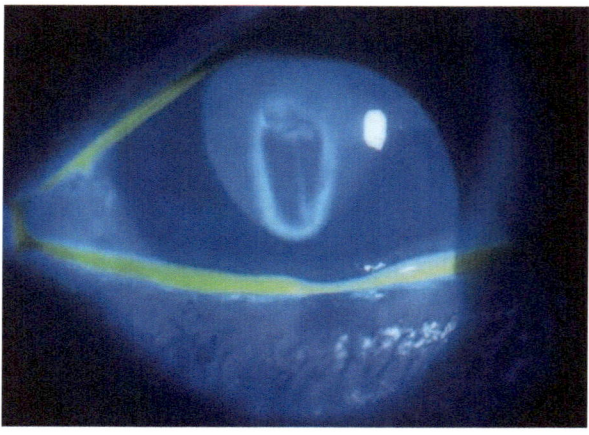

Fig. 10.2 Blood layering in the anterior chamber, defining hyphema. (© 2022 American Academy of Ophthalmology)

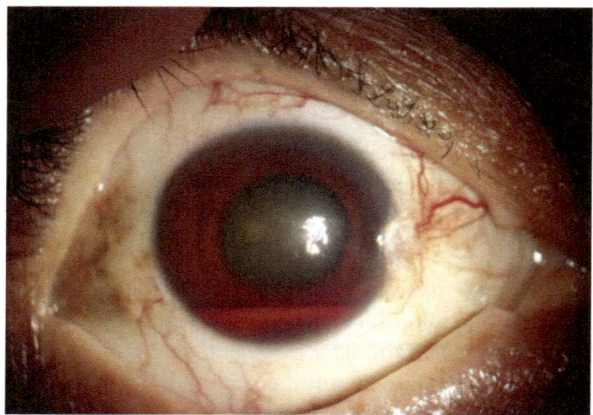

(resting on the forehead and upper cheek) to protect the eye from further injury until surgery can be performed. Administer IV antibiotics (typically moxifloxacin or vancomycin and ceftazidime).

- *Closed globe injuries:* Even if there is no open globe injury, there can still be significant trauma to the intraocular structures. Patients may endorse visual changes and exhibit decreased vision, photosensitivity, and ocular pain. Below are descriptions of some specific conditions of closed globe trauma.

  - *Traumatic hyphema:* Suspect if the patient exhibits blood in the anterior chamber. Take care to measure intraocular pressure, as it can be elevated. Manage with topical steroids and cycloplegics to lower the intraocular pressure and stabilize the iris to minimize the risk of rebleeding. Counsel the patient to avoid activities that will put strain on the eye or agitate settled blood products and to protect the eye with a rigid barrier. Anti-platelet and anticoagulants should be avoided if possible (Fig. 10.2).

- *Traumatic iris injury:* Suspect if the patient exhibits a poorly reactive pupil. The pupil may be mydriatic, miotic, or irregularly shaped (corectopia). Iridodialysis (disinsertion of the peripheral iris from the wall of the eye) may occur and hyphema is also common.
- *Traumatic iritis:* Suspect in patients that endorse pain and photosensitivity typically within 24 h of blunt traumatic injury to the eye or orbit. There is usually anterior chamber cell and scleral injection along with mydriasis or miosis. Manage with topical steroids and cycloplegics.
- *Corneal abrasion:* Patients typically exhibit pain, photophobia, tearing. A discrete area of fluorescein staining on the cornea is diagnostic. Manage with topical antibiotics and lubricants (e.g., erythromycin ointment). Topical cycloplegic agents can also help with pain control.
- *Corneal foreign body:* Patients present similarly to those with corneal abrasions but a foreign body is identified on examination. Always consider the possibility of an intraocular foreign body and rule out open globe injury. Superficial foreign bodies can be removed using a 30-gauge needle. Once removed the patient can be managed similarly to patients with corneal abrasions.
- *Chemical injuries:* Patients exhibit pain, injection, and sometimes severe damage to the cornea, conjunctiva, and adnexal structures. While the eye is often markedly injected after a chemical insult very severe injuries may present without injection (white eye) due to destruction of the conjunctival blood vessels and blanching of the ocular surface. Basic agents are more damaging than acidic agents, but regardless of the agent the first priority is to irrigate with normal saline until the pH of the ocular surface is physiologic (7–7.5). After physiologic pH is achieved patients are managed with topical antibiotics, lubricants, steroids, and cycloplegics. Intraocular pressure may be elevated, requiring topical pressure-lowering drops. Cases with severe damage to the cornea and/or conjunctiva patients may require amniotic membrane placement.
- *Posterior segment pathology:* Patients will typically endorse floaters, blurred and decreased vision, or photopsias (e.g., flashing lights). A dilated fundus exam should be performed emergently to rule out the presence of traumatic cataract, vitreous hemorrhage, retinal detachment, choroidal rupture, and other possible injuries.

Cellulitis [3]

Inflammation of the periorbital and orbital tissues are common reasons for emergency room presentations in ophthalmology. The inflammation is most commonly due to bacterial infections but can also be due to viral or fungal infections or, in rarer instances, due to autoimmune disease, malignancy, or foreign bodies. The periorbital and orbital soft tissue are composed of multiple layers. Arranged from superficial to deep these layers are the skin, orbicularis muscle, and orbital septum. Deep to the septum is the orbit proper which is predominantly comprised of fat and extraocular muscles. Inflammation limited to the layers superficial to the orbital septum defines pre-septal cellulitis, and inflammation that penetrates the orbital septum defines orbital cellulitis. It is important to distinguish if the inflammation is pre-septal or orbital, as these are managed differently. Imaging, most commonly CT Orbits with contrast, can be helpful in identifying post-septal inflammatory changes.

Selected Diagnoses

- *Orbital cellulitis*: Orbital cellulitis (Fig. 10.3) refers to the spread of infection or inflammation deep to the orbital septum. As a result, orbital tissues such as the fat, extraocular muscles, globe, and the optic nerve can become inflamed. As a result, these patients will exhibit "orbital signs" including limited eye movement and pain with eye movements. If severe, the patient may exhibit decreased color vision, decreased visual acuity, high intraocular pressure, and a relative afferent pupillary defect. Most commonly, orbital cellulitis arises from an extension of sinusitis. Other etiologies include spread from pre-septal cellulitis, dacryocystitis, dacryoadenitis, oral infection, direct trauma, and less commonly hematogenous spread. Management involves early blood cultures, a complete blood count, and a metabolic panel. Erythromycin sedimentation rate and C-reactive protein levels may be obtained if there is concern for necrotizing fasciitis. Admission for inpatient monitoring and initiation of broad spectrum intravenous antibiotics is

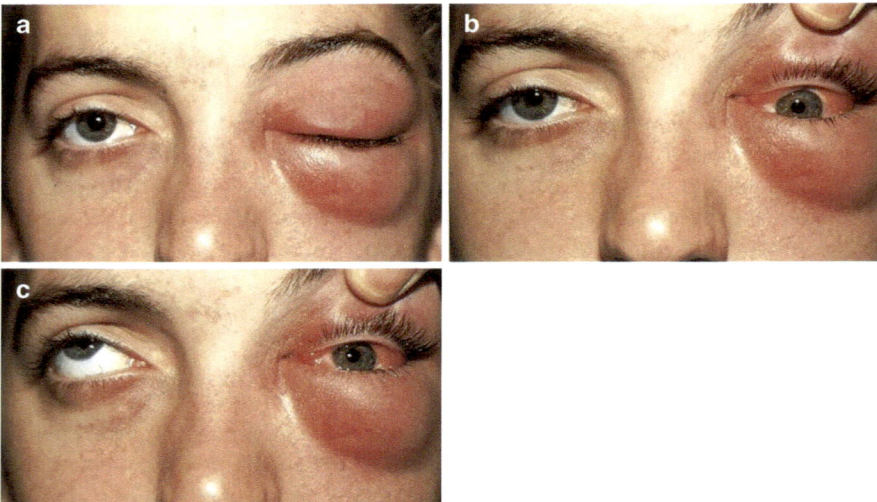

Fig. 10.3 Orbital cellulitis: (**a**) periorbital swelling; (**b**) chemosis and inferior displacement of the eye in primary gaze; (**c**) limitation in supraduction. (© 2022 American Academy of Ophthalmology)

indicated. Antibiotics are narrowed as the patient improves clinically or when a specific pathogen is identified. Surgical intervention may be required in cases where an orbital or subperiosteal abscess develops, or if there is evidence of optic nerve compromise (e.g., afferent pupillary deficit, decreasing vision). If the intraocular pressure is severely elevated patients may require an urgent canthotomy and cantholysis. The presence of optic nerve compromise indicates a guarded prognosis.

- *Pre-septal cellulitis:* Pre-septal cellulitis tends to present with periorbital edema and erythema but by definition does not involve the post-septal orbital tissues. The patient will exhibit normal vision, color vision, eye movements, and pupil responses. Chemosis and injection are mild in most cases. Pre-septal cellulitis often responds promptly to antibiotic therapy and oral antibiotics usually are sufficient in reliable patients. If there is no improvement with oral antibiotics, intravenous antibiotics may be considered. If an abscess develops, incision and drainage are indicated and often will speed recovery. Young children and infants warrant close observation and possibly admission as the risk of progression to orbital cellulitis is higher in this age group due to the underdeveloped orbital septum. Prognosis is good but can become guarded if development of orbital cellulitis occurs.
- *Necrotizing Fasciitis:* Highly virulent pathogens such as Streptococcus and *Methicillin-resistant Staphylococcus Aureus* (MRSA) can lead to a necrotizing soft tissue infection of both pre-septal and orbital tissues. These cases require broad spectrum antibiotics and emergent surgical debridement of infected and non-viable tissues. Periorbital necrotizing fasciitis is associated with a slightly better prognosis than similar infections of other regions but remains a vision and life-threatening entity requiring prompt recognition and intervention.

High Eye Pressure [6]

Intraocular pressure is considered a vital sign of the eye. It should always be measured as a part of an emergent ophthalmic assessment. Elevated intraocular pressure is considered to be greater than 21 mmHg although this pressure is not necessarily vision threatening. Patients with severely elevated eye pressure commonly present with eye pain, redness, and decreased vision from optic neuropathy or corneal edema. The differential diagnosis of elevated intraocular pressure is vast, and it is important to perform a complete eye exam to determine the etiology. Common etiologies of acutely elevated eye pressure are listed below.

Selected Diagnoses

- *Acute Angle Closure:* Acute angle closure occurs when there is apposition of the peripheral iris and cornea preventing flow of fluid through the trabecular meshwork. This may occur when aqueous fluid produced behind the iris is unable to travel anteriorly through the pupil. A build-up of fluid behind the iris pushes the iris anteriorly closing the angle structures and causes a dramatic increase in intraocular pressure. These changes can occur in the setting of an enlarged lens (i.e., cataract), a small eye, or a combination of the two. Less common causes of acute angle closure include traumatic lens dislocation and medication side effect (i.e., topiramate).

- *Chronic Angle Closure Glaucoma*: Patients with chronic angle closure accumulate scar tissue between the iris and trabecular meshwork over time. This is most commonly due to chronic apposition of the iris near the trabecular meshwork. Alternatively scar tissue can be formed secondary to intraocular inflammation (i.e., uveitis), trauma, or post-surgical changes. Similar to acute angle closure, the intraocular fluid is unable to drain from the eye, leading to elevated eye pressure.
- *Neovascular Glaucoma*: Neovascular glaucoma develops when underlying ischemia of the ocular tissues results in the formation of a network of blood vessels on the iris in the area of the trabecular meshwork. This process can lead to bleeding, inflammation, and scarring and eventual occlusion of the meshwork. Patients with neovascular glaucoma often have other significant ischemic comorbidities, such as diabetes, hypertension, hyperlipidemia, or systemic vascular disease.
- *Uveitis:* Some forms of anterior uveitis cause a secondarily elevated intraocular pressure due to inflammation of the trabecular meshwork.
- *Hyphema:* See Trauma section.
- *Orbital compartment syndrome*: See Trauma section.

Treatment

- Determination of the underlying etiology of the elevated intraocular pressure is critical.
- Medical therapies are the mainstay of treatment. Topical (timolol, dorzolamide), oral (acetazolamide), and intravenous therapies to decrease aqueous production and increase aqueous outflow can decrease the intraocular pressure. Osmotic agents, such as glycerin or mannitol, can also be useful in acutely decreasing the intraocular pressure. These agents must be used judiciously in patients with uncontrolled hypertension, diabetes, or heart failure.
- Laser peripheral iridotomy (LPI) uses focused light to reestablish the trans-iris flow of aqueous humor and is indicated in cases where the high eye pressure is caused by pupillary block from lens-iris apposition.
- Incisional surgical intervention may be required if medical therapy or LPI fails to lower intraocular pressure.

Prognosis

- Elevated intraocular pressure of any etiology can cause severe damage to the optic nerve head and permanent vision loss. The prognosis is dependent on the magnitude and duration of pressure elevation and as a result pressure should be controlled as quickly as possible.

The Red Eye [7–9]

A chief complaint of a "red eye" is a common cause for presentation to emergency rooms and clinics. Although this is a term used colloquially, "red eye" refers to hyperemia or injection of any part of the eye or its immediate surrounding structures. These structures include the conjunctiva, episclera, and sclera. While the etiology is often benign and self-limiting, it is important to recognize vision-threatening cases. Diagnosis and treatment are often predicated on the exam and accurate recognition of the specific location of the hyperemia.

Anatomy of the Red Eye

- Fundamentally hyperemia is the result of engorgement of superficial blood vessels which impart a red hue to the overlying tissue.
- This process can occur in the conjunctiva, episclera, sclera, or adnexal structures (e.g., eyelids) and is commonly referred to as conjunctivitis, episcleritis, scleritis, and stye/chalazion/blepharitis, respectively.
- Extravasation of blood from the vessels is not technically hyperemia but may also present with a red eye. Bleeding often occurs in the potential space between the conjunctiva and the sclera (subconjunctival hemorrhage).

History Taking

- Begin with a series of open-ended questions to allow the patient a chance to express what brought the symptoms to their attention and how the symptoms presented.
- Determine the acuity of the presentation and whether there have been prior episodes.

- Elicit additional symptoms, such as discharge, photophobia, floaters, or decreased vision.
- Identify relevant ocular history, such as uveitis or contact lens use.
- Identify other relevant medical history, such as rheumatologic disease (often associated with uveitis, scleritis, and episcleritis).

Physical Examination

- Begin by measuring visual acuity, intraocular pressure, and observing pupillary response to light.
- Observe the eye without magnification or the use of the slit lamp. This gross examination best detects the violaceous hue of scleritis, an important diagnosis not to miss.
- Perform biomicroscopic examination using a slit lamp to further localize the hyperemia. It can be helpful to apply anesthetic drops to a cotton swap and then attempting to gently move the conjunctiva while watching to see if the hyperemic tissue displaces with the swab—suggesting conjunctival hyperemia over scleral hyperemia.
- Carefully scan for any discharge. Note the character (mucopurulent, serous) and quantity of this discharge.
- Inspect the cornea for edema, opacities, and foreign bodies.
- Examine the anterior chamber, paying attention to the depth of the chamber and presence of free-floating debris, blood, cell, or flare.
- ***Additional Exam Techniques*** [7]

  - ***Fluorescein:*** Fluorescein dye can identify corneal epithelial defects seen in corneal abrasions, as well as in bacterial, viral, and neurotrophic keratitis.
  - ***Topical 2.5% Phenylephrine:*** This simple test can be extremely helpful to determine the depth of the hyperemia. Instill a drop of 2.5% phenylephrine and then wait a few minutes. Phenylephrine drops will improve conjunctival hyperemia and often lead to full resolution of episcleral hyperemia within 10–15 min (a unique feature) and will have minimal effect on scleral hyperemia. Note: phenylephrine will induce dilation of the pupil and can exacerbate acute angle closure glaucoma and should therefore be avoided if there is strong suspicion of this diagnosis.
  - ***Topical Anesthetics:*** The patient's response to topical anesthetic drops can be helpful in differentiating the irritated red eye. Discomfort associated with corneal abrasions or corneal ulcers is significantly reduced, whereas the discomfort associated with scleritis or uveitis typically persists.

Selected Diagnoses [7–9]

The differential diagnosis for the red eye is broad. Below is a list of the most common causes in order of decreasing prevalence.

- **Dry Eye** (10,000–61,000/100,000 person-years): Patients often exhibit irritation that improves with lubrication and examination may reveal punctate epithelial erosions. Manage with improved lubrication of the ocular surface.
- **Blepharitis** (1800–3100/100,000 person-years): Patients may exhibit eyelid erythema or telangiectasias, crusting or matting, or even swelling such as in hordeolum or chalazion.
- **Conjunctivitis** (1100–1500/100,000 person-years): Patients exhibit conjunctival hyperemia associated with discharge. Conjunctivitis can be due to several etiologies:
    - **Allergic:** Often associated with itching and other allergy symptoms, watery discharge, and papillary conjunctival reaction. Manage with topical antihistamines, topical steroids, cold compresses, and improved lubrication.
    - **Viral:** Often associated with recent cold symptoms, regional lymphadenopathy (e.g., preauricular lymphadenopathy), watery discharge, and conjunctival follicular reaction. If severe, patients may have pseudomembranes and corneal epithelial defects. Manage with frequent lubrication with preservative-free artificial tears and cold compresses. Viral conjunctivitis is highly contagious so proper personal protective equipment should be worn throughout the exam and the patient should be counselled on isolation from others and frequent hand hygiene to prevent spread.
    - **Bacterial:** Discharge is typically thick and purulent and is accompanied by a papillary conjunctival reaction. Topical antibiotics may be prescribed but are often not necessarily, as this condition is often self-limited. A notable etiology is gonococcal conjunctivitis which is described as hyperpurulent and can be associated with rapid corneal ulceration. Treatment of gonococcal conjunctivitis involves frequent ocular lavage with normal saline to clear the purulence, topical antibiotics, and systemic treatment with ceftriaxone. Sexual partners should be notified and screened.
    - **Chlamydial:** In contrast to other causes of bacterial conjunctivitis, chlamydial conjunctivitis is associated with follicular conjunctival reaction. Manage with systemic antibiotics against chlamydia (e.g., azithromycin) and topical antibiotics. Coinfection with gonorrhea should be ruled out.

- **Episcleritis** (70/100,000 person-years): Patients exhibit hyperemia that improves with topical phenylephrine, and symptoms are generally mild. Episcleritis is rarely associated with systemic disease. Manage with topical lubrication, topical non-steroidal anti-inflammatory medications, or topical steroids.
- **Scleritis:** Patients often endorse unilateral boring periorbital or retrobulbar pain. Examination is notable for hyperemia that does not improve with topical phenylephrine. Under diffuse lighting (e.g., room lights) the hyperemia may appear as a violaceous hue. Importantly, scleritis is associated frequently with systemic rheumatologic diseases, such as granulomatosis with polyangiitis, so a detailed review of systems is critical. Manage with oral non-steroidal anti-inflammatory medications or steroids (make sure to prescribe proton pump inhibitors to prevent stomach ulcers).

- *Microbial Keratitis:* Otherwise known as a corneal ulcer, this condition is often associated with severe eye pain (except in neurotrophic ulcers) and photophobia. Examination may reveal a corneal epithelial defect with underlying corneal opacity (if bacterial or fungal) or a superficial dendritic lesion (if viral). Obtain samples to send for culture and Gram stain, or polymerase chain reaction tests. Manage with topical antimicrobials depending on the suspected etiology.
- *Acute Anterior Uveitis (Iridocyclitis):* Patients exhibit pain, photophobia, and examination reveals anterior chamber flare, cell, fibrin, or endothelial keratic precipitates. It can be associated with systemic rheumatologic disease. Treatment generally involves topical steroids and cycloplegics.
- *Endophthalmitis:* Endophthalmitis refers to an infection inside the eye, which can be bacterial, viral, or fungal. It is often associated with significant vision loss and pain. Treatment includes intravitreal antimicrobials and less commonly surgery.
- *Acute Angle Closure Glaucoma:* See High Eye Pressure section.

Flashes and Floaters [4, 5, 10]

Visual disturbances such as photopsias (i.e., flashing lights) or dark spots floating through the visual field can be very disturbing for patients and a reason for an emergent presentation to a healthcare provider. Patients presenting with these symptoms patients warrant dilated fundus examination for careful evaluation of the posterior segment, including the vitreous, retina, and optic nerve. The following are common conditions that cause flashes and floaters.

Selected Diagnoses

- *Vitreous syneresis:* As the vitreous ages, it degenerates from a jelly-like substance to a liquid (syneresis). This process is often experienced by patients as the formation of black spots that move across in the visual field ("floaters"). Simple floaters from syneresis alone are benign and require no treatment but can be bothersome to the patient.
- *Posterior Vitreous Detachment:* In its normal state, the vitreous is connected to the retina via adhesions at the optic nerve and ora serrata. A posterior vitreous detachment refers to the process of the vitreous detaching from the retina. It is commonly an age-related change but can also be associated with trauma or after surgery. Patients often notice a new large floating dark spot in the vision and may have photopsias as well. The classic physical exam finding is a Weiss ring, a mobile crescentic opacity visible in the posterior vitreous, which represents the condensed vitreous that was attached to the edges of the optic disc. An isolated posterior vitreous detachment is benign with no visual sequela; however, poste-

rior vitreous detachments may be complicated by vitreous hemorrhage a retinal tear or retinal detachment.

- **Retinal tear/break:** The retina is a thin sheet of neural tissue. When it is pulled, torn, or broken, patients may notice photopsias as the neural tissue is stimulated. The photopsias are often accompanied by floaters. When left unrecognized or untreated, retinal tears can lead to a retinal detachment, thus prompt recognition and treatment is critical. Treatment usually consists of applying laser burns to the retina surrounding the break, thus isolating the tear to prevent progression towards a retinal detachment.
- **Retinal detachment:** A retinal detachment occurs when the retina is separated from its attachments to the outer wall of the eye. This can occur if there is a break in the retina and fluid travels through the tear beneath the retina (rhegmatogenous retinal detachment). Alternatively inflammatory fluid may exudate from leaky vessels in the choroid and build-up under the retina (serous retinal detachment). Finally, tissue within the vitreous may pull the retina off the wall of the eye (tractional retinal detachment). Patients will typically endorse a dark shadow, bubble, or severely blurred vision in a section of the visual field. The visual field by confrontation may be limited in the section corresponding to the detached portion of the retina. Treatment of retinal detachment depends on the etiology but may require surgical intervention if rhegmatogenous or tractional in nature. Anti-inflammatory medications (e.g., steroids) may be appropriate in cases of serous detachment. When surgical intervention is appropriate, the status (attached or detached) of the macula is helpful in determining the urgency of the surgery. If the macula is attached, surgery is generally considered more urgent so that the macula does not become detached.
- **Vitreous hemorrhage:** Bleeding inside the vitreous cavity often causes numerous floaters in the visual field—patients may even describe seeing red blood in the visual field. Vitreous hemorrhage can occur after eye trauma, in patients with proliferative retinopathy (e.g., diabetic retinopathy), or after a posterior vitreous detachment. Often, the retina cannot be visualized when the hemorrhage is dense and B-scan ultrasonography is needed to determine if the retina is attached. If there is no tear or retinal detachment, the patient can be observed closely while the blood clears. Surgery is indicated if there is a retinal detachment, if there is suspicion for a retinal tear, or if the blood has not cleared after several months.
- **Migraine with aura:** The photopsias produced in auras are typically colorful and described as a circular "kaleidoscope" that expands over time. Generally, these phenomena will last for no more than 30 min.
- **Uveitis:** Posterior segment inflammation can cause patients to see floaters. There are a vast number of possible etiologies of this inflammation, including infections such as syphilis, tuberculosis, herpes viruses, and bacterial endophthalmitis.
- **Neoplasm:** Neoplasms of the posterior segment such as malignant melanoma, lymphoma, or retinoblastoma can cause both flashes and floaters. An intraocular mass may be visualized on exam or on B-scan ultrasonography.

References

1. Vaziri K, Schwartz SG, Flynn HW, Kishor KS, Moshfeghi AA. Eye-related emergency department visits in the United States, 2010. Ophthalmology. 2016;123(4):917–9.
2. Weisenthal RW, Daly MK, de Freitas D, Feder RS, Orlin SE, Tu EY, Van Meter WS, Verdier DD. External disease and cornea. San Francisco: American Academy of Ophthalmology; 2019.
3. Korn BS, Burkat CN, Carter KD, Perry JD, Setabutr P, Steele EA, Vagefi MR. Oculofacial plastic and orbital surgery. San Francisco: American Academy of Ophthalmology; 2019.
4. Bhatti MT, Biousse V, Bose S, Danesh-Meyer HV, Falardeau J, Levin LA, Phillips PH, Williams ZR. Neuro-ophthalmology. San Francisco: American Academy of Ophthalmology; 2019.
5. McCannel CA, Berrocal AM, Holder GE, Kim SJ, Leonard BC, Rosen RB, Spaide RF, Sun JK. Retina and vitreous. San Francisco: American Academy of Ophthalmology; 2019.
6. Girkin CA, Bhorade AM, Crowston JG, Giaconi JA, Medeiros FA, Sit AJ, Tanna AP. Glaucoma. San Francisco: American Academy of Ophthalmology; 2019.
7. Gilani CJ, Yang A, Yonkers M, Boysen-Osborn M. Differentiating urgent and emergent causes of acute red eye for the emergency physician. West J Emerg Med. 2017;18(3):509–17.
8. Leibowitz HM. The red eye. N Engl J Med. 2000;343(5):345–51.
9. Robinson B, Acorn CJM, Millar CC, Lyle WM. The prevalence of selected ocular diseases and conditions. Optom Vis Sci. 1997;74(2):79–91.
10. Sen HN, Albini TA, Burkholder BM, Dahr SS, Dodds EM, Leveque TK, Smith WM, Vasconcelos-Santos DV. Uveitis and ocular inflammation. San Francisco: American Academy of Ophthalmology; 2019.

Index

GPSR Compliance

The European Union's (EU) General Product Safety Regulation (GPSR) is a set of rules that requires consumer products to be safe and our obligations to ensure this.

If you have any concerns about our products, you can contact us on ProductSafety@springernature.com

In case Publisher is established outside the EU, the EU authorized representative is:

Springer Nature Customer Service Center GmbH
Europaplatz 3
69115 Heidelberg, Germany

Batch number: 09204675

Printed by Printforce, the Netherlands